ENDOGENOUS NEUROPROTECTION

ENDOGENOUS NEUROPROTECTION

BERNHARD J. SCHALLER

Nova Biomedical Books
New York

For permission to use material from this book please contact us:
Telephone 631-231-7269; Fax 631-231-8175
Web Site: http://www.novapublishers.com

Library of Congress Cataloging-in-Publication Data

Schaller, Bernhard.
Endogenous neuroprotection / Bernhard J. Schaller.
p. ; cm
Includes bibliographical references and index.
ISBN: 978-1-60456-228-6 (hardcover)
1. Cerebral ischemia—Prevention. 2. Cerebral anoxia. I. Title.
[DNLM: 1. Brain Ischemia—physiopatholgy. 2. Ischemic Attack, Transient—physiopathology.
WL 355 S298e 2008]
RC388.5.S33 2008
616.8'1—dc22

2007052757

Published by Nova Science Publishers, Inc. ✦ New York

In Memoriam

"Das Bewusstsein eines erfüllten Lebens und die Erinnerung an viele gute Stunden sind das größte Glück auf Erden"

Marcus Tullius Cicero (106 BC-43BC)

In memoriam to my father

Contents

Main Abbreviations

ADP	adenosine diphosphate
AMPA	α-amino-5-hydroxy-3-methyl-4-isoxazole propionic acid
AP	activator proteins
ASA	acetylsalicylic acid
ATP	adenosine triphosphate
BBB	blood brain barrier
BCL	B-cell-lymphoma
Ca^{2+}	calcium
CBF	cerebral blood flow
CMRGLC/CMRO2	cerebral metabolic rate of glucose/cerebral metabolic rate of oxygen
CREB	camp-response-element-binding protein
CRE	camp-response element
DAG	diacylglycerol
DNA	deoxyribose nucleic acid
DOG	1,2 dioctanoyl-rac-glycerol
Epo	erythropoietin
GABA	gamma aminobutyric acid
GLUT-1	glucose-transporter-1
GPCR	G-protein coupled receptors
GSK	glycogen synthase kinase
HIF-1	hypoxia inducible factor-1
HMG-CoA	3-hydroxy-3-methylglutaryl-CoA
Hsp	heat shock protein
ICAM	intercellular adhesion molecule
IL-1	interleukin-1
iNOS	inducible nitric oxide synthase
K^+	potassium
K_{ATP}	ATP-sensitive K^+channels
LPS	lipopolysaccaride
MAP-kinase	mitogen-activated protein kinase
MCA	middle cerebral artery

MGLURs	metabotropic glutamate receptors
MMPs	Matrix metalloproteinases
mRNA	messenger ribonucleic acid
MnSOD	manganese superoxide dismutase
NFκB	nuclear-factor κB
NAALADase	*N*-acetylated alpha-linked acidic dipeptidase (
NMDA	N-methyl-D-aspartate
NO	nitric oxide
NO^-	nitroxyl anion
Na^+	sodium
O_2	oxygen
PAI-1	plasminogen activator inhibitor-1
PARP	poly(ADPribose) polymerase
PET	positron emission tomography
pH	power of hydrogen
PKC	protein kinase C
PLA_2/C/D	phospholipase A_2/C/D
PMA	phorbol 12-myristate 13-acetate
RNS	reactive nitrogen species
ROS	reactive oxygen species
R(-)-PIA	N6-(R)-phenylisopropyladenosine
tPA	tissue plasminogen activator
sEPOR	serum erythropoietin receptor
SPT	8-Sulphophenyl theophylline
SRC	v-src sarcoma (Schmidt-Ruppin A-2) viral oncogene homolog (avian)
TIA	transient ischemic attack
TNF	tumor necrosis factor
VEGF	vascular endothelial growth factor

Abstract

Background: Neurons can be pre- and also postconditioned by various procedures to resist subsequent ischemic events. Such a preconditioning mechanism induced is characterized by a brief episode of ischemia that renders the brain more resistant against subsequent longer ischemic events. This phenomenon of ischemic tolerance has been shown in different experimental model organisms of cerebral ischemia and recently also in few human studies. The basic molecular mechanisms of ischemic tolerance remain largely unknown in detail until present, but are initiated over several hours or days, and can persist for up to a week ore more. Preconditioning can be induced by short bouts of ischemia, several pharmaceutical substances (e.g. adenosine analoga) and volatile anesthetics all imposed before the index ischemic events. A brief ischemia of an organ other than the brain can likewise initiate cerebral ischemic tolerance, which has been called „remote preconditioning". According to the recent literature, short ischemic events after an index ischemia can also initiate ischemic tolerance in the brain, especially leading to (*i*) improved post-ischemic endothelial function, (*ii*) reduced infarct size and (*iii*) less apoptosis; this (neuro)protective maneuver has been called „postconditioning". In this context, nothing is yet know wheather "postconditioning" has significant clinical relevance in the brain. In the present study, the hypothesis was therefore tested if postconditioning lessens ischemic injury in the brain of an animal model with clinical relevance. Special reference is given to molecular imaging methods to visualize cerebral metabolism and blood flow changes.

Methods: Different experimental models in the cat have yet been developed to examine the mechanisms responsible for changes after cerebral ischemia. Middle cerebral artery occlusion (MCAO) model in the cat is best established in this context, and therefore used and modified in the present study. To better analyze the outcome in this animal model, the cats were therefore divided into two subgroups: (*i*) one <u>without</u> prior MCAO ("*hemicraniectomy in normal brain*") and (*ii*) one <u>with</u> prior MCAO ("*decompressive hemicraniectomy after MCA occlusion*") before performing left-sided hemicraniectomy. Regional cerebral blood flow (CBF), cerebral metabolic rate of oxygen (CMRO2) and of glucose (CMRGLC) were measured by positron emission tomographie (PET) studies from the brain tissue underneath the craniectomy at 2, 20 and 28 hours after hemicraniectomy.

Results: In the subgroup with *hemicraniectomy in normal brain*, CBF significantly decreased and oxygen extraction fraction (OEF) significantly increased after operation as compared to the operative procedure. But, CMRO2 and CMRGLC decreased only in regions with most severe CBF reduction. These effects remained for at least a day after the operative procedure irrespective of corrective sustaining cranioplasty. In the subgroup with *decompressive hemicraniectomy after MCAO*, 30% of the animals showed pronounced recovery of CBF in parts of the ischemic territory that lasted until the next day after the operation.

Conclusion: Our animal model is effective in studying cerebral postconditioning as induced by decompressive hemicraniectomy. In the present study performed with help of molecualr imaging by PET, there was found for the first time that postconditioning significantly reduces ischemic cerebral damage in a clinical relevant animal model. The effect of recovery of the CBF in the *decompressive hemicraniectomy after MCAO* subgroup is beyond the effect of the expansion of the brain as demonstrated by the corrective sustaining cranioplasty in a part of the animals and can therefore related to a postconditioning effect. Altogether these new imaging insights into the molecular mechanism of cerebral ischemic tolerance open a new window to the future discovery of potentially useful (pharmacological) targets for acute neuroprotection as well as preventive therapy in stroke. The clinical potential to visualize such neuroprotective strategies may extend beyond cerebral ischemic tolerance to include other brain injury states as well.

Keywords: cerebral ischemia – ischemic tolerance – preconditioning – postconditioning - apoptosis – neuronal death.

Chapter 1

1. Introduction

Stroke is the third leading cause of death in the highly industrial countries. Ischemic stroke counts for 80 % of the cases, as the brain is more vulnerable to ischemic events than any other organ system. Brief interruption of cerebral blood flow (CBF) for only 5 minutes already leads to neuronal death in corresponding brain regions, whereas only 20-40 minutes of ischemia is required to achieve cell death for example in cardiac myocytes or kidney cells (Lee et al., 2000). This extraordinary vulnerability of the brain tissue to ischemic damage reflects its high metabolic rate, varying in different brain regions (Rosner et al,. 1986). Although the human brain represents only about 2.5% of the body weight, it accounts for 25% of basal metabolism, a metabolic rate 3.5 times higher than in other primate species (Lee et al., 2000). In addition, central neurons depend almost exclusively on glucose as energy substrate, and brain stores of glucose are limited. However, energy substrate limitations are not solely responsible for the brain's high vulnerability to ischemia. Rather, it appears that the brain's intrinsic cell-to-cell and intracellular signaling mechanisms, normally responsible for information processing, become harmful under ischemic cell death in all tissues, including free radical production, activation of catabolic enzymes, membrane failure, apoptosis and inflammation (Calabresi et al., 2000).

In transient ischemic events, two different pathophysiological processes contribute to the evolution of infarction: the initiation of infarction during the ischemia phase and the reversion or maturation of the infarction during the ischemia phase and the reversion of maturation of the infarction process during the recirculation phase. In the initial phase, oxygen extraction fraction increases in regions with severely reduced CBF (Graf et al., 1996). In experimental animal studies of 30 minutes vessel occlusion, this may be sufficient to salvage the brain tissue over such rather short ischemic episodes (Graf et al., 1996). From this point of view, processes during the recirculation phase depend largely on the initiation, i.e. magnitude and duration CBF reduction and the viability of the altered brain tissue. However, practically any stimulus capable of causing damage to a tissue or organ can, when applied close to (but below) the threshold of damage, activate endogenous protective mechanisms – thus potentially lessening the impact of subsequent, more severe stimuli. The penumbra concept has been extended in recent years by including ischemic alterations of various electrophysiological and biochemical variables as markers for functional performances

(Astrup et al., 1981; Heiss, 1992). From earlier work, it is evident, that the penumbra has a temporal dimension in that it is not only a function of the severity of the perfusional disturbances but also of its duration (Heiss et al., 1976). This relationship and, in addition, secondary mechanisms extending the ischemic vascular territory make the penumbra a dynamic process propagating from the most severely ischemic core to regions in the periphery of vascular territories with impaired perfusion (Strong et al., 1983; Heiss et al., 1994). This is even more so after recanalization of the occluded vessel, which may be beneficial if the time point of reperfusion is early, but also if substantial tissue compartments are still viable because of sufficient residual blood supply (Heiss et al., 1983). At present, the only therapy demonstrated to improve outcome from acute ischemic stroke is thrombolysis of the clot responsible for the ischemic event (Higashida et al., 2003). Accordingly, stroke patients treated by thrombolysis, have better chance of survival with little or no residual disability, but at the same time they may suffer the consequences of a reperfusion damage. In order to minimize the damage caused by the exposure to this insult, the protocol for the thrombolysis treatment should include simultaneous administration of neuroprotective compounds (Schaller et al., 2004). Furthermore, finding of long-acting neuroprotective compounds could enable preventive administration of such drugs to stroke-prone subjects. The development of potent neuroprotective compounds depends on elucidation of neuroprotective mechanisms, enabling to focus on specific targets conferring maximal neuroprotection (Reshef et al., 2000) with the long-term goal of allowing therapeutic augmentation of the endogenous neuroprotective mechanisms in cerebral ischemia and possibly development of new neuroprotective strategies for ischemic stroke treatment (Blanco et al., 2006). However, these broad-spectrum approaches also made clear that preventing neuronal death and thus reducing neurological damage are complex tasks that cannot be successfully resolved by targeting single mechanisms. One of the most promising approaches is to create ischemic tolerance in the brain represent the use of pharmacological preconditioning paradigms.

Preischemic functional state and the level of metabolism are among factors determining the susceptibility of central neurons to ischemic events. It has been shown that brief subletal cerebral ischemia induces tolerance of neurons to subsequent more prolonged lethal ischemia (Dowden et al., 1999). This phenomenon was defined as ischemic tolerance. The exitotoxic hypothesis of ischemic neuronal death is based on neurotoxic effects of high extracellular concentrations of glutamate that result in enhanced excitatory synaptic activity. This toxicity is largely related to glutamate mediated calcium influx into affected nerve cells (Kristian et al., 1998). Brief non-lethal ischemia does not reach the critical level for initiation of neuronal death but produces, on contrary, acquired tolerance to subsequent lethal ischemia (Shimazaki et al., 1998). In such „ischemia-tolerant“ neurons, intracellular calcium elevation is markedly inhibited after an anoxic-aglycemic episode, as compared to neurons in control (Shimizaki et al., 1998).

Chapter 2

2. Review of the Literature

2.1. Definition of Ischemic Tolerance

Preischemic functional state and the level of metabolism are among factors determining the susceptibility of neurons to ischemia (Ferriero, 2005). It has been shown that brief, sublethal cerebral ischemia induces tolerance of neurons to subsequent more prolonged lethal ischemia (Dowden et al., 1999). This phenomenon is called ischemic preconditioning and represents probably a fundamental cell/organ response to certain types or levels of injury (Ettaiche et al., 2001). Analysis of the determinants of infract size that may be effected by this neuroprotective maneuver showed that this phenomenon was independent of differences in oxygen supply during ischemia, as the regional collateral blood flow in the preconditioned and the unpreconditioned brain was comparable. Establishing this protective phenotype in response to stress depends on a coordinated response at the genomic, molecular, cellular and tissue levels (Schaller et al., 2002; Gidday, 2006).

Cerebral ischemic tolerance can be established by global and focal ischemia, both of which are capable of protecting the other form of ischemia (Chen J et al., 1997). In addition, cerebral ischemic tolerant states have been induced by chemical, pharmacological, electrical and/or anoxic/ischemic means (cited in Schaller et al., 2002). Further experiments have shown that metabolic and physical stresses can also induce cross-tolerance to cerebral ischemia, but the protection by cross-tolerance is relatively modest (Kirino, 2002). In most of these states of ischemic tolerance, the neuronal protection requires several days to develop. In exceptional cases, effective tolerance may be achieved only after 12 to 15 days.

Ischemic tolerance was first described in the heart (Reimer et al., 1986; Swain et al., 1984), and has since been seen in a variety of other organ systems (Hawaleshaka et al., 1998), including the brain. In the heart, it has become apparent that brief ischemia provides a marked increase in myocardial resistance to a later ischemic event that would be lethal otherwise (Tomai et al., 1999). Murray et al. (Murray et al., 1986) found that four periods of 4-minute coronary occlusion, each separated by 5 minutes of reperfusion, led to a reduction in infarct size produced by a subsequent 40-minute occlusion of the coronary artery. The called this method of enhancing ischemic tolerance in the heart "preconditioning". Extensive research in experimental animals has provided data on the potential mechanism of ischemic preconditioning in the heart, which includes adenosine receptor activation, opening of mitochondrial Adenosine triphosphate (ATP)-sensitive potassium channels, and production of endogenous protective stress proteins.

Cerebral ischemic tolerance was first demonstrated by use of a global ischemic model (Kitigawa et al., 1990; Kitigawa et al., 1991), where two minutes of transient ischemia were required to provide protection against global cerebral ischemia 24 hours later. Ischemic tolerance in the brain seems to be markedly different from that found in the heart: the temporal profile of its onset and duration suggests divergent mechanisms (Chen et al., 1996). The brief onset and duration of tolerance in the much longer time frame required for induction of tolerance in brain and its persistence over days is more compatible with the idea of newly induced protein synthesis as basic mechanism. Cerebral ischemic tolerance can be established by global and focal ischemia, both of which are capable of protecting the other form of ischemia (Kitigawa et al., 1990; Kitigawa et al., 1991). The underlying mechanism of cerebral ischemic tolerance still is not fully understood. It seems that two distinct phases are involved (Kirino, 2002; Schaller et al., 2002). Firstly, a cellular defense function against ischemia may be developed by the mechanisms inherent to neurons such as posttranslational modification of proteins or expression of new proteins via a signal transduction system to the nucleus (Reshef et al., 2000). Secondly, a stress response and synthesis of stress proteins (heat shock proteins) may be activated. These mechanisms are mediated by chaperones by unfolding misfolded cellular proteins and helping the cell to dispose of unneeded denatured proteins (Trendelenburg et al., 2005).

Preconditioning has been observed in virtually all species and models tested in animal studies, as well as in humans, and are touted as the "gold standard" by which all other neuroprotective strategies are judged.

2.2. Pathophysiology of Focal Cerebral Ischemia

2.2.1. The Core and Penumbral Regions of Cerebral Infarction

There are two major categories of experimental ischemia: (*i*) global hypoxia and/or ischemia models and (*ii*) focal ischemia models. In global hypoxia and/or ischemia models, typically two or four cervical vessels to the brain are temporarily interrupted and circulation restored after some delay. In focal ischemia models, the middle cerebral artery (MCA) is typically occluded either permanently or temporarily to allow reperfusion (Kanemitsu et al. 2002).

Herein, the focus will be given on the pathophysiology of brain cell death in focal ischemia models because human ischemic stroke is best modeled with both permanent and reperfusion models of stroke. Following typical embolic vascular occlusion in humans, there is spontaneous thrombolysis and spontaneous recanalization that occurs but at variable times following initial occlusion. Angiographic controlled studies in humans have shown that spontaneous recanalization can occur around 17% of the time within the first 6 to 8 hours of stroke and that approximately half of the vessels will reopen in 3 to 4 days (Kassem-Moussa et al., 2002). In animal models of focal MCA occlusion, the volume of cerebral infarction becomes equal to that of permanent MCA occlusion when temporary MCA recanalization is allowed beyond 2 to 3 hours. Therefore, in most cases, human MCA occlusion is probably best modeled with permanent cerebral ischemia models. Because the current basis of emergent stroke treatment is vessel recanalization however, both permanent and reperfusion models are relevant for human stroke therapy.

Brain injury and neuronal death necessitates at least 1 to 2 minutes of focal vascular occlusion. In animal models, CBF is most greatly reduced in a central region of brain (infarct "core") and in a graded fashion centrifugally from the core ("penumbra") (see Figure 1). CBF decreases to less than 15% of baseline within the core, which leads to reductions in adenosine triphosphate (ATP) levels to 25% of baseline. CBF decreases to between 15% and 40% by definition in penumbral regions, and ATP levels decrease to between 50% and 70% of control within minutes of vessel occlusion. All neurons within the core region will infarct despite experiencing an increase in ATP levels to two-thirds of normal and return of normal oxygen partial pressure if the duration of ischemia is 30 minutes or more (Smith, 2004). Some neurons within the penumbra will die as well; as the duration of focal ischemia lengthens, the size of the infarct will increase so that after 2 to 3 hours of focal ischemia in rodents, the size of the infarct will be equal to that found with permanent vascular occlusion (see Figure 2). The process by which the penumbra is destroyed represent the focus of most ischemia research, as prevention of this infarct growth with intervention would be expected to salvage neuronal tissue. Several strategies are successful for protecting against penumbral destruction, fostering the concept of "neuroprotection".

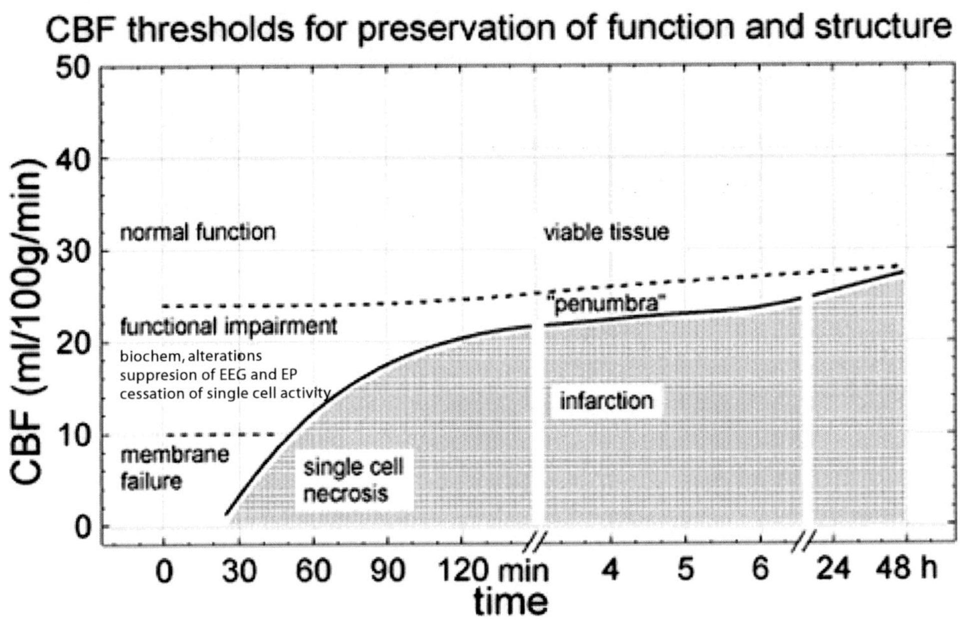

Figure 1. Diagram of cerebral blood flow (CBF) thresholds required for the preservation of function and morphology of brain tissue. The development of single cell necrosis and infarction is dependent on the duration of time for which CBF is impaired below a certain level. The solid line separates structurally damaged from functionally impaired but morphologically intact tissue (the "penumbra"), and the dashed line distinguishes viable from functionally impaired tissue (with permission of WD Heiss, Germany).

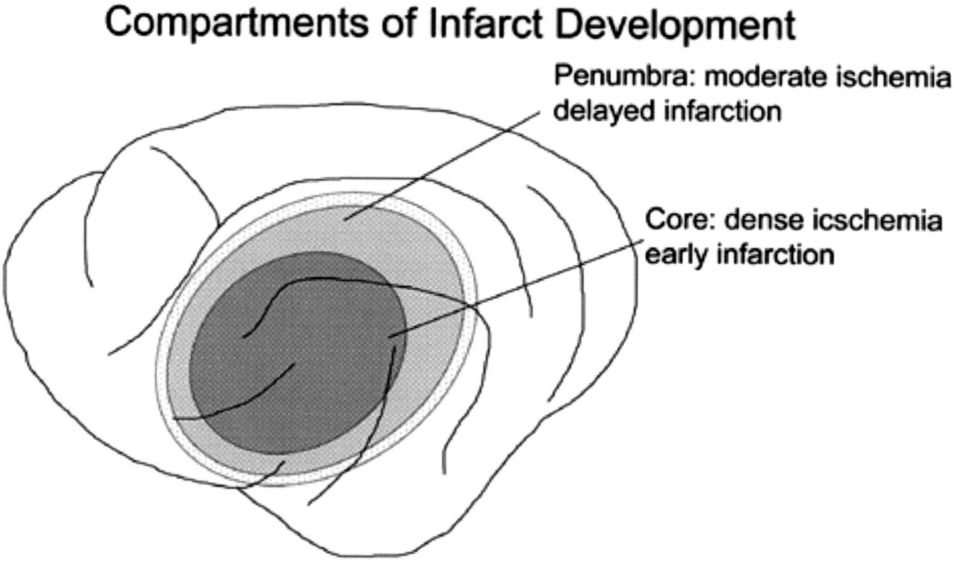

Figure 2. Diagram of ischemic area distinguishing between dense ischemia in the core and moderate ischemia in the penumbra (with permission of WD Heiss, Germany).

Cells die by means of two major methods: (*i*) necrosis and (*ii*) apoptosis. Necrotic cell death is an energy-passive process independent of protein synthesis that is characterized by loss of cellular architecture and ultimately culminates in cytoskeletal breakdown, with edema formation within 12 to 24 hours of ischemia. The morphologic features of apoptotic cell death are quite different, with deoxyribose nucleic acid (DNA) laddering and regular clumping of chromatin (apoptotic bodies) (Smith, 2004). This is followed by a stereotypical loss of cellular architecture (which takes several days) that involves the activity of caspases (family of cysteine proteases) and other enzyme systems. Necrotic cell death is more common with more extreme levels of ischemia, whereas apoptotic cell death is more common with less severe insults. Thus, the core tissue of an infarct dies with a necrotic process, and, depending on the location within the penumbra, cells die by means of either method, with apoptosis more common for cells further away from the core.

2.2.2. Process of Cerebral Infarction and Cellular Death

Within minutes of vascular occlusion, brain tissue is deprived of glucose and oxygen and the acidic byproducts of metabolism accumulate. Although the exact sequence of events is debatable, what follows is a likely sequence of events responsible for the early damage to neurons. This loss of substrate and decrease in power of hydrogen (pH) level leads to cessation of the electron transport chain activity within mitochondria, which results in a rapid decline in ATP concentration. Loss of ATP leads to failure of the sodium (Na^+)/potassium (K^+)-ATPase, which results in a marked intracellular increase in intracellular Na^+ concentration (Smith, 2004). Persistent depolarization allows calcium (Ca^{2+}) entry, and higher intracellular Na^+ levels reduce the efficacy of the $2Na^+$-Ca^{2+} symport, which further increases intracellular Ca^{2+}. Because the membrane potential reaches the electrical threshold for discharge, neurons inside the core infarct exhibit ischemic discharges whereby they fire repetitively, releasing their transmitters locally and at distant targets (Smith, 2004). These ischemic depolarizations further exacerbate energy needs.

A high intracellular Ca^{2+} level initiates several events, including activation of calpain protease activity that effects the structural integrity of both the intra- and extracellular structure and phospholipase activity that degrades cellular membranes. Increased Ca^{2+} also induces nitric oxide synthase activity and expression, which favors the formation of peroxynitrate. Nitric oxide is a physiological messenger in the central nervous system that if formed from L-arginine in a reaction catalyzed by the NO synthase (Moro et al., 2005; Rodrigo et al., 2005). Nitric oxide reacts with superoxide to from peroxynitrite (Moro et al., 2005; Rodrigo et al., 2005) that is a highly reactive free radical species.

The resulting influx of Ca^{2+} damages the mitochondria, which further exacerbates energy failure. Mitochondrial damage occurs in part by means of direct Ca^{2+} toxicity as mitochondria attempt to sequester Ca^{2+}. This eventually overwhelms the mitochondria, which leads to mitochondrial depolarization and swelling. In isolated brain mitochondria, 2-5% of the electron flow leak in the form of superoxide and hydrogen peroxide (Baza et al., 1998). Hyodrogen peroxide is also the precursor of reactive hydroxyl radical. As an additional mechanism of damage, the mitochondrial transition pore is opened by high Ca^{2+} levels, free radicals, and Ca^{2+}-dependent calpain activity, which allows mitochondria to release mitochondrial ions and cytochromes - most important cytochrome C - into the cytoplasmatic cytochrome C release likely initiates apoptosis. Mitochondria also produce free radicals that are toxic both to the mitochondria and the cell as a whole, especially if sufficient oxygen is present as during reperfusion.

The amount of cellular damage is highly dependent on the tissue glucose concentration. Perhaps paradoxically, the volume of brain infarction is markedly increased when the tissue glucose level exceeds 16 to 20 mmol/L. This is likely a pH effect as an oversupply of glucose in the setting of oxygen deficit enhances glycolysis, which further reduces the pH level. Hyperglycemia in human stroke is associated with infarct expansion (Parsons et al., 2002) and worse neurologic outcome (Bruno et al., 2002).

Depending on the degree of ischemia and its duration, the above events may be minimal and short-lived, resulting in only temporary cellular dysfunction (see Figure 3). This is the likely cause of transient ischemic attacks (TIA) in which neurologic dysfunction is apparent but full recovery is the rule. For more severe levels of ischemia (i.e., less collateral blood flow) and more sudden decline in CBF (embolic as opposed to thrombotic), the chemical cascade released owing to ischemia will overcome cellular homeostasis and lead to cellular death. The highly reactive radicals damage the cells by several mechanism including lipid peroxidation, tyrosine nitration, sulfhydril oxidation and nitroslyation and DNA breakage (Freeman et al., 1982; Kehrer et al., 1993). Recent studies also demonstrate that these radicals inhibit the mitochondrial respiratory chain and involve in the apoptotic cell death through cytochrome c mediated pathway (Lo et al., 2003). The initiation and execution phases of apoptosis are both dependent on caspases, the cytosolic cysteine proteases that are responsible for the proteolytic cleavage of many intracellular proteins, resulting in the morphological and biochemical changes associated with apoptosis.

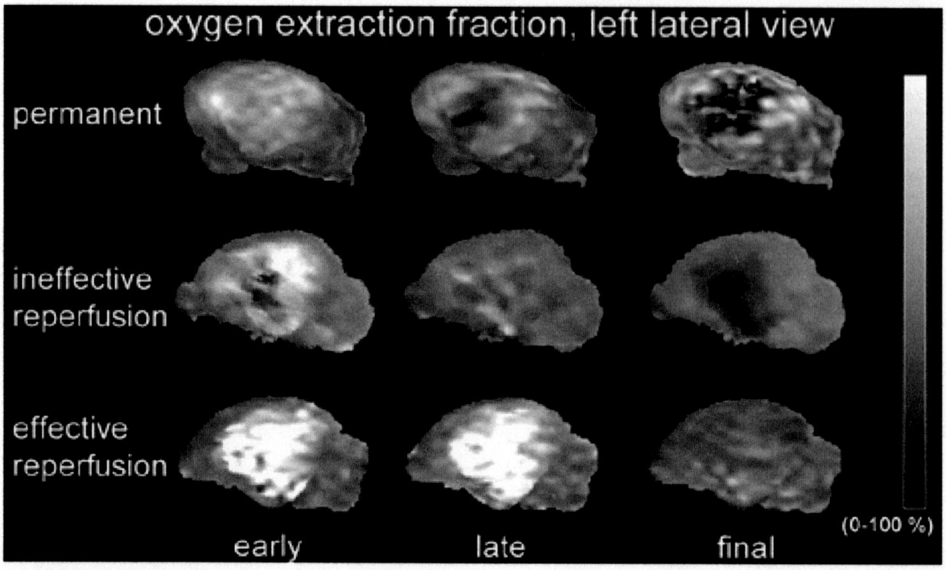

Figure 3. Reconstructed surface view of left hemispheric oxygen extraction fraction (OEF) in three cats after permanent or transient occlusion of the middle cerebral artery. Increased OEF indicates penumbra tissue, decreased OEF identifies irreversible tissue damage.Centrifugal conversion of penumbra into irreversible damage in permanent occlusion, reperfusion can only reverse penumbra and prevent damage as long as increased OEF indicates tissue viability (with permission of WD Heiss, Germany).

Neurons within the ischemic core die exclusively by means of a necrotic mechanism initiated and propagated by the mechanisms reviewed earlier. Damage within the penumbra is mediated by different mechanisms. Because ATP levels and CBF magnitude are only marginally reduced within the penumbra, there is insufficient ischemia to directly cause the cataclysmic processes that happen so quickly within the core. Important insight into the mechanism of penumbral infarction came from the discovery that blockade of the glutamate receptor mitigated penumbral damage and reduced infarct size (Simon et al. 1984). Glutamate levels within the core and penumbra increase rapidly in ischemia, likely due to synaptic release from core neurons undergoing ischemic depolarization but also directly from cells damaged by ischemia. Glutamate agonizes the *N*-methyl-d-aspartate (NMDA) receptor, a Ca^{2+} membrane channel, which increases Ca^{2+} influx to the cell. Glutamate also agonizes the amino-hydroxy-methyl-isoxalone propionic acid (AMPA)/kainate receptor, which allows both Na^{+} and Ca^{+} entry, and the metabotropic receptor (quisqualate), which increases intracellular cyclic adenosine monophosphate levels, altering protein kinase activity, proteolysis, and lipolysis. Iontophoresis of glutamate, a glutamate agonist, causes immediate injury to cerebral neurons, and glutamate levels within experimental ischemic brain can reach levels sufficient to be toxic (Lipton, 1999). This increase in glutamate is bimodal in focal ischemia, increasing within 1 to 2 minutes of ischemia but also after several hours. NMDA-receptor competitive and noncompetitive antagonists can reduce experimental infarct volume as much as 30%–50% (Lipton, 1999). NMDA-receptor antagonists are effective for mitigating damage during this early window of time and are most effective if present within tissue before the induction of ischemia.

Ischemic depolarization of core neurons results in a centrifugal release of glutamate into the penumbra, which leads to direct toxicity of penumbral neurons (Hossmann, 1994). This may lead to a sufficient increase in intracellular Ca^{2+} levels to be directly toxic to penumbral neurons or, if insufficient, allow these neurons to recover function over time. The cascade of events in the core, however, produces a diffusible cadre of K^{+}, free radicals, and glutamate that can directly damage penumbral neurons.

It is important that free radical production is enhanced within penumbral tissue during reperfusion, and this may account for much of the damage seen in the penumbra (Lipton, 1999). Free radicals are produced in high concentration from partially damaged mitochondria that are exposed to oxygen. Spin-trap free radical inhibitors and uric acid can dramatically reduce infarct volume in reperfusion models, which supports the contribution of free radical damage in reperfusion (Sydserff et al., 2002; Marshall et al., 2001; Yu et al., 1998). In addition, moderate increases in intracellular Ca^{2+} lead to induction of inducible nitric oxide (NO) and subsequent peroxynitrate production, so free radical generation can be delayed and prolonged, leading to secondary damage to neurons hours to days later. Free radicals convert the unsaturated lipids to radical species that both damage membrane lipid and propagate free radical generation. Phospholipase A_2 is activated by lipid peroxidation and degrades membrane lipid, which leads to direct membrane breakdown and loss of fluidity. Free radicals also directly affect proteins, especially membrane channels leading to exacerbation of high intracellular Ca^{2+} and inhibition of mitochondria respiratory chain enzymes. Peroxynitrate and other free radial species produce single-strand DNA breaks within penumbral regions during reperfusion. These breaks induce poly (adenosine diphosphate ribose) polymerase (PARP), a nuclear enzyme that repairs single-strand breaks. PARP activity is fueled by a reduction in nicotinamide-adenine dinucleotide, and it is hypothesized that marked increases in PARP activity deplete the reduced form of nicotinamide-adenine dinucleotide, contributing to cellular energy failure (Lipton, 1999). PARP inhibition, or knockout of PARP, markedly reduces infarct volume in reperfusion models but has no effect on permanent ischemia, which supports the role of free radicals in reperfusion injury.

Sublethal injury to neurons favors initiation of apoptosis, causing cells within the penumbra to die by means of this pathway rather than the necrotic pathway, depending on the magnitude of initial injury. How apoptosis is initiated is unclear, but two major contributors are increased cytosolic cytochrome C, which is released through the mitochondrial permeability transition pore from injured mitochondria, and calpain activity from increased intracellular Ca^{2+} concentration. Cytochrome C induces caspase activity, a major apoptotic enzyme system, setting forth the complex, likely irreversible process of apoptosis. Cells undergoing apoptotic cell death exhibit regular, rounded regions of nuclear chromatin clumping followed by formation of apoptotic bodies that contain cytoplasm and clumped chromatin. DNA double-stand breaks occur and DNA laddering is seen. This contrasts with free radical–induced single-strand DNA breaks that induce PARP activity and lead to necrotic cell death. As opposed to necrotic death, cellular cytoplasm does not become eosinophilic and the cells simply appear to shrink; there is no surrounding edema.

A hallmark distinction between necrotic cell death and apoptosis is that energy and protein synthesis are necessary for the latter to proceed (Du et al., 1996). Because apoptosis requires further gene transcription and protein synthesis, there must be some integrity of the nucleus and gene transcription processes. This may account for the differential pathways selected for cell death depending on location within the core or penumbra. Another remarkable feature of apoptosis is the time between ischemic insult and eventual death of the neuron. Depending on the severity and duration of ischemia, apoptotic cell death does not begin until the 3rd day and can extend as far as 2 weeks. It is interesting that although the process is inexorable once initiated, it can be halted with proteases. It can be prevented altogether with mild hypothermia (35°C) during the early stages of ischemia, which suggests a potential therapeutic role for hypothermia in penumbra salvage (Edwards et al., 1995). Conversely, the process is accelerated by hyperthermia, as are necrotic processes.

Finally, ischemia also damages the brain's capillaries and endothelium and incites an inflammatory response whereby white blood cells infiltrate regions of infarct. The contribution of white blood cells to the process of secondary damage is controversial (Emerich et al., 2002), but white blood cells (chiefly neutrophils) appear within the infarct within 24 hours, at the appropriate time to cause damage (see Figure 4).

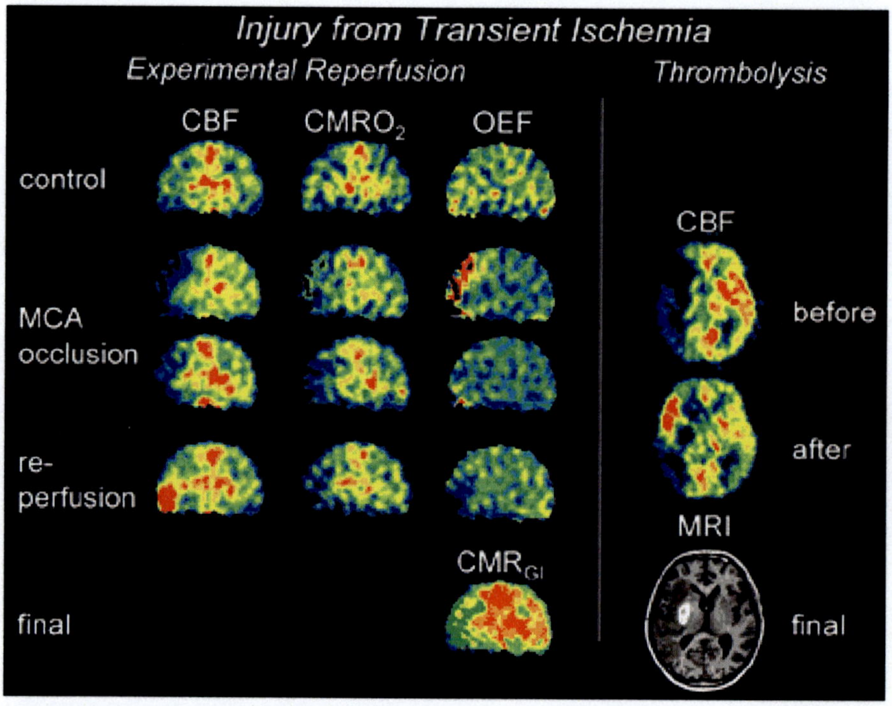

Figure 4. Left side: sequential PET images from an individual cat undergoing 60-min MCAO and reperfusion resulting in an unfavorable outcome. Images represent CBF, CMR2, and OEF before (control), immediately after and 30 min after MCAO, and after reperfusion. During the ischemic episode, CMRO2 deteriorated further and the initially increased OEF decreased already during ischemia. After reperfusion, pronounced hyperperfusion occurred in this particular cat, and final CMRglc showed major deficits. Right side: patient study demonstrating only partially successful reperfusion after thrombolysis (frontal part of ischemic focus), resulting, however, in pronounced hyperperfusion. Structural damage as determined by MRI occurred in this particular case in both nonreperfused and hyperperfused portions of the ischemic territory (with permission of WD Heiss, Germany).

In addition, the prevention of leukocyte accumulation (by blocking cytokines, blocking adhesion molecules like intracellular adhesion molecule 1, or depleting leukocytes) reduces the experimental infarct size - especially in reperfusion models. Neutrophils are neurotoxic in several ways, including generation of free radicals from nicotinamide adenine dinucleotide phosphate oxidase, NO production from inducible NO synthase (NOS) within neutrophils, and formation of arachidonic acid leading to more free radical formation. It does not appear that intravascular sludging by white blood cells exacerbates ischemia (Lipton, 1999).

Cerebral tissue can protect itself from repeated ischemic insults (see Figure 5). A rat brain exposed to transient MCA occlusion will be protected against ischemic cell death within the conditioned zone after several days and lasting up to 7 days (Kirino, 2002). Preconditioned cells will develop initial morphologic changes of early ischemia but will later recover. This ischemic tolerance of brain is likely mediated by the induction of protective genes, including heat-shock protein and B-cell lymphoma (BCL)-2 (protein involved in the apoptosis pathway), and an increased ability of cells to sequester intracellular Ca^{2+}. This process may have teleologic importance and can potentially offer a neuroprotective avenue.

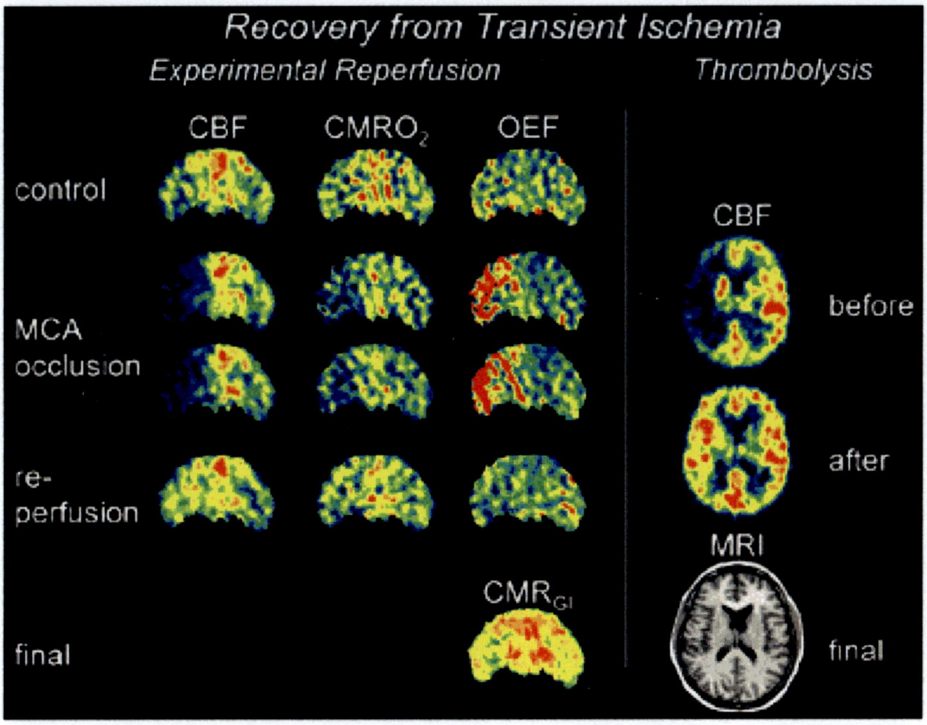

Figure 5. Left side: sequential PET images from an individual cat undergoing 60-min MCAO and reperfusion resulting in a favorable outcome. Images represent CBF, CMRO2 and OEF before (control), immediately after and at the end of MCAO and after reperfusion. During the ischemic episode, CMRO2 did not deteriorate further and OEF remained increased. Hyperperfusion was not pronounced in this particular cat, and final CMRglc did not show major deficits. Right side: patient study demonstrating successful reperfusion after thrombolysis. Structural damage as determined by MRI did not occur in this particular case (with permission of WD Heiss, Germany).

2.3. Ischemic Tolerance as an Archetypical Non-Specific Stress Response

Stroke, ischemic preconditioning, and ischemic preconditioning plus stroke all induce gene changes that overlap little among conditions (Stenzel-Poore et al., 2004; Schaller et al., 2003). Stroke induce robust up-regulation of gene expression whereas preconditioning followed by stroke results in a marked down-regulation. Genes up-regulated by stroke suggest activation of stress/inflammatory pathways and increased metabolism and ion channel function (Stenzel-Poore et al., 2004). Preconditioning tends to decrease genes involved in these pathways. Follow-up experiments show that preconditioning decreased voltage-gated potassium currents in vitro and increased bleeding time (Stenzel-Poore et al., 2004). Preconditioning reprograms the response to ischemic injury via transcriptional changes that may suppress metabolic pathways and immune responses, reduce ion channel activity, and decrease blood coagulation (Stenzel-Poore et al., 2004). These changes resemble evolutionarily conserved responses to decreased blood flow and oxygen availability that occur during hibernation (Stenzel-Poore et al., 2004).

The interaction of severity and duration of oxygen deprivation and the development of (irreversible) cell-damage is highly variable in different species but all animals have developed specific strategies to cope with restricted substrate delivery. Accordingly, invertebrates were increasingly used as animal model to study ischemic tolerance (Haddad et al., 2001). Although it is unlikely that inducible protection against ischemic events is an evolutionary advantage, it is likely that (physiological) mechanisms that protect against global hypoxia can also protect against ischemia.

Adapting to extreme habitats, a variety of vertebrates have developed strategies to tolerate prolonged stages of brain anoxia (anoxia tolerance) or reduced cerebral perfusion and capacity to deliver oxygen during hibernation. Anoxia- tolerant species are instructive about the pathophysiological adaptations that occur in the central nervous system for them to survive an anoxic or hypoxic-ischemic event. Answering the question of (*i*) how the brain tissue of these animals induces and sustains tolerance to hypoxia, and (*ii*) how these animals actively remerge from the anoxic/ischemic state and cope with reoxygenation, could help to identify novel strategies to enhance or prolong the survival of ischemic neurons under ischemic circumstances. Anoxia tolerance and hibernation have multiple independent evolutionary origins, even with single species (Hochachka et al., 2001). Given the differences in habitat, anatomy, physiology and phylogeny, it is not surprising that different animals have evolved different strategies to cope with anoxia and severe reductions in nutrient perfusion. However, some common key mechanisms, of differing relevance in the various species, have been identified: (*i*) suppression or arrest of metabolism (Storey et al., 1990), (*ii*) regulation of key glycolytic enzymes (Lutz et al., 1997), (*iii*) reduction in the conductance of ion channels (ion-flux arrest) (Gentile et al., 1996; Igelmund et al.), (*iv*) suppression of neural activity (Spangenberger et al., 1995), (*v*) expression of chaperons (Chang et al., 2000), (*vi*) adaptation in blood rheologhy (Frerichs et al., 1994) and (*vii*) expression and accumulation of antioxidants (Rice et al., 2002). Under conditions of anoxia/ischemia in hibernating animal's brain cells, ATP demand decreases drastically. Specifically, protein synthesis and degradation decrease to 10% of normoxic rates, and urea and glucose biosynthesis decrease to zero. Decreases in the energy demands of the Na^+/K^+-ATPase are less than for overall ATP turnover. Thus, during periods of hypoxia/ischemia, in some types, the Na^+/K^+-ATPase becomes the cell's dominant energy sink, accounting for up to 75% of the ATP demand of the cell (Golden et al., 2001). Interestingly, in the brain where under normoxic conditions Na^+/K^+-ATPase function is required to maintain ionic gradients and membrane potential, compensation for hypoxia includes not only a decrease in Na^+/K^+-ATPase function, but also a decrease in membrane ion permeability (Rego et al., 2001). These changes in membrane ion permeability permit the anoxic brain of hibernating animals to maintain an electrochemical potential while decreasing the energy demands on the Na^+/K^+-ATPase. From this point of view, ischemic tolerance and hibernation appear to involve at least partially similar mechanisms.

2.4. Experimental Models of Ischemic Tolerance

A large number of animal models studies of cerebral ischemia have demonstrated that brief periods of non-lethal focal or global ischemia may have a protective effect against further episodes of brain ischemia. To differentiate between experimental phenomena and potential clinical relevance, the choice of the experimental model is of obvious importance according to ischemic tolerance stimulus and subsequent lethal ischemia. In the following, we tried therefore to group the animal models into: (*i*) global-global ischemia, (*ii*) focal-global ischamia, (*iii*) global-focal ischemia and (*iv*) focal-focal ischamia. The advantage of these models are that they allow reproducing cerebral ischemia under standard conditions.

2.5. Animal Models of Cerebral Ischemic Tolerance

2.5.1. Global-Global Ischemia Animal Model

The first experimental reports demonstrating cerebral ischemic tolerance were performed in a gerbil-model and used brief periods of global ischemia followed by reperfusion to protect against subsequent prolonged global ischemia (Kitagawa et al., 1999; Kirino et al., 1991; Kato et al., 1991). There is experimental evidence in the study of Kitigawa et al. (Kitigawa et al., 1991) that 2 minutes, but not 1 minute of ischemic preconditioning was followed by ischemic tolerance in the brain and that a 24-hour, but not a 12-hour, interval was necessary for induction of such a tolerance. This induced cerebral ischemic tolerance persisted for at least 2 days (Kitigawa et al., 1991). As in the myocardial cells, multiple brief ischemic episodes induced more potentially cerebral ischemic tolerance than a single episodes (Kitigawa et al., 1991). These observations in global ischemia demonstrated selective protection of CA1 hippocampal neurons in up to 90% of the cells (Kitigawa et al., 1991). As seen in review of the respective literature, cerebral protection achieved by brief global ischemia ranges between 20-91%. It relates to infarct size and does not show any differences between varying animal species (see table 1). The variability may rather derive from the different intervals between the preconditioning ischemic episode and subsequent lethal ischemia. The definition of the exact duration of cerebral ischemia and the interhemispheric interval, both of which are relevant for induction of tolerance, may be critical, as increased glutamate release and accelerated ischemic brain tissue damage have been reported after repeated episodes of global ischemia in a rat model (Lin et al., 1992). It seems that brief episodes of sublethal cerebral ischemia may be beneficial in the setting of subsequent ischemic events, whereas more prolonged or continuous preexposure beyond the tolerance threshold may exacerbate ischemic damage (Corbett et al., 1997; Paratt et al., 1994). Subtle differences seem to exist in the ability of aged versus young animals to tolerate ischemia.

2.5.2. Focal-Global Ischemia Animal Model

In the cortical region of rat forebrain, Galzier et al. (Galzier et al., 1994) reported that subsequent global ischemic cell-tissue damage (induced by bilateral carotid occlusion and systemic hypotension) was diminished after a time-period of 20 minutes of distal MCA occlusion followed by 24 hours of reperfusion. In addition, focal ischemia was able to induce cerebral protection in ipsilateral hippocampal neurons outside the original brain tissue of initial focal ischemia (see table 2) (Miyashita et al., 1994). Non-lethal ischemia can induce mild gliosis in rat hippocampus (particularly in the hilus) and cerebral cortex. Such activation of astrocytes involves induction of stress proteins in these neurons, such as heat shock proteins (Currie et al., 2000), thus enhancing astroglial functions and increasing the ability of these cells to capture glutamate and maintain water ion homeostasis (Valentim et al., 2001). Since dephosphorylated heat shock proteins act as chaperons and protect other proteins from denaturation (Guo et al., 2000), the down-regulation of heat shock protein phosphoryltion observed in the dentate gyrus after preconditioning may contribute to the maintenance of normal astrocytic function. However, the interaction of several stress proteins may be much more important than the level of specific heat shock protein for neurolal survival after ischemic events, because recent studies emphasized the crucial role of the interactions of several stress proteins for molecular chaperon activity (Glover et al., 1998). Molecular chaperons have been defined as proteins that bind to and stabilize an otherwise unstable conformer of another protein. By controlling binding and release, they participate in the folding and assembly of nascent and unfolded peptides and facilitate protein transport to a particular subcellular compartment and disposal by degradation (Hartl et al., 1996).

2.5.3. Global-Focal Ischemia Animal Model

The possible clinical relevance of ischemic tolerance to focal ischemia is related to the experimental phenomenon that preceding brief periods of global ischemia decrease the infarct volume in rats following permanent medial cerebral artery occlusion (Simon et al., 1993).

Table 1. Ischemic tolerance after global ischemia in selected studies (modified from Weih et al., 2001)

Author	Species	Pre-con	Intervall	Ischemia	Outcome	Method	Protection [1)]
Perez-Pinzon et al. 1997	rat	2 min CCAO and hypotension	0.5 h	10 min CCAO	3.7 d	CA1	70-91%
Kitigawa et al. 1990	gerbil	2x2 min CCAO	24 h	5 min CCAO	7 d	CA1	53-98%
Kobayashi et al. 1995	rat	2x2 M KCl	24 h	6 min	6 d	necrosis	56%
Heurteaux et al. 1995	rat	3 min CCAO	72 h	6 min CCAO	1-7 d	CA1	90%
Dowden et al. 1999	gerbil	2x1.5 min CCAO	72 h	5 min CCAO	10,30,60 d	CA1	20-89%

Legend. pre-con: preconditioning; min: minutes; CCAO: common carotid artery occlusion; M: moles; KCl: potassium chloride; h: hour; d: day; CA1: measurement of neuronal density of the hippocampal CA1 section.

[1)] related to the size of infarction.

Table 2. Ischemic tolerance after focal ischemia in selected studies (modified from Weih et al., 2001)

Author	Species	Pre-con	Intervall	Ischemia	Outcome	Protection [1)]
Toyoda et al. 1997	rat	20 min CCAO/MCAO	24 h	60 min	48 h	41-61%
Matsushima et al. 1995	rat	global/MCAO	96 h	MCAO	96 h	66%
Wiegand et al. 1999	rat	3-NPA i.p	12 h,	90 min MCAO	72 h	35-70%
			1,2,3,7 d			
Stagliano et al. 1999	rat	1-3x 55 min MCAO	30 min	1 h, 24 h	24 h	33-39%

Legend. pre-con: preconditioning; min: minutes; CCAO: common carotid artery occlusion; MCAO: middle cerebral artery occlusion;3-NPA: 3-nitropropionic acid; i.p.: intraperitonal; h: hour; d: day.

[1)] related to the size of infarction.

Table 3. Ischemic tolerance in vitro models in selected studies (modified from Weih et al., 2001)

Author	Species	Pre-con	Intervall	Ischemia	Outcome	Protection [1)]
Bruer et al. 1997	rat: cortical neurons	90 min OGD	24,48,72 h	180 min OGD	4,24,48 h	6-72%
Khaspekov et al. 1998	rat: hippocampal culture	60 min OGD	24 h	90 min	24 h	40-60%
Grabb et al.1999	mice: mixed culture	5-30 min OGD, K^+; NMDA	7,24,72 h	120-150 min OGD	24 h	30-50%
Weih et al. 1999	rat: cortical neurons	120 min, 3-NPA	24-48 h	120-150 min OGD	24 h	30-70%
Kasischke et al. 1999	mice: hippocampal slice	1 h 3-NPA	1 h	15 min OGD	45 min	50%

Legend. pre-con: preconditioning; min: minutes; h: hour; OGD: oxygen-glucose deprivation; K+: potassium; NMDA: N-methyl d-aspartate; 3-NPA: 3-Nitropropionic acid.

[1)] related to LDH measurement.

Simon et al. (Simon et al., 1993) demonstrated that a 48-hour-, but not a 24-hour-interval between global ischemia and MCA occlusion was required for successful induction of ischemic tolerance. The ischemic tolerance phenomenon may be relevant not only to glial or vascular cells but also to neurons, as cerebral infarction involves necrosis affecting both neuronal and non-neuronal tissue (Chen et al., 1997). Although all cell types in the brain tissue are capable of expressing stress proteins, these results further demonstrate distinct patterns of expression of individual proteins, e.g. heat shock proteins, in response to a given ischemic event (Geddes et al., 1996). But the precise mechanism of transcription would need further clarification.

2.5.4. Focal-Focal Ischemia Animal Model

TIA, as demonstrated clinically, represent an analogous effect to the experimental tolerance to focal ischemia induced by prior exposure to transient focal ischemia. Experimentally, optimal conditions have been established for ischemic tolerance induction by sublethal focal ischemia in rats (see table 2); (*i*) the time interval necessary for development of tolerance, and (*ii*) the duration of induced tolerance to a second more prolonged focal ischemic challenge (Chen et al., 1996). Thirty minutes of transient focal ischemic preconditioning by single or divided stimulus was found to represent the optimal prerequisite for ischemic tolerance induction lowed of resulting in 30% reduction of infarct volumes. Ischemic tolerance could not be demonstrated one day after ischemic preconditioning but was seen first the second day lasting 5-7 days after induction. The protection of brain tissue after cerebral preconditioning was not only limited to neurons but also extended to non-neuronal tissue as mentioned above. CBF assessed by ^{14}C-iodantipyrine in the tolerant cortex was not increased above control either before or during the ischemic challenge resulting in infarction. For this reason, the mechanism of ischemic tolerance cannot be attributed to CBF alterations. This is in accordance with an another animal study, that used more severe transient focal ischemia (180 minutes) and resulted only in increased CBF in the ischemic region, but ischemic tolerance could not be demonstrated after a second ischemic event 4 days later (Matsushima et al., 1995). For this reason, it is generally accepted that CBF cannot explain neuroprotection inducing ischemic tolerance. However, the timing of protection from subsequent neurological deficits might be related to the different profiles of protection from infarction observed across the brain after induced ischemic tolerance (Barone et al., 1998): Ischemic preconditioning that induced brain protection in rats was more pronounced in the cortical area leading to hindlimb deficits than in the area leading to forelimb deficits. Perhaps other factors, such as increased nervous system plasticity after cellular damage, are also involved in protection from neurological deficits in preconditioning induced ischemic tolerance. These results underline that ischemic tolerance is not associated with systematic but most probably with regional/local release of neuroprotective factors.

2.6. *In Vitro* Models of Cerebral Ischemic Tolerance

Germanisov et al. (Germanisov et al., 2001) were able to demonstrate preconditioning by motor activity induces a significant, though short-lasting protection of hippocampal neurons against ischemia. It markedly improves the ability of pyramidal neurons to recover somatic excitability and synaptic transmission following prolonged global (decapitation) ischemia (see table 3). Such protection is dramatic even after 90 minutes decapitation ischemia at 30°C and may be related to changes in cell metabolism (reduction of oxygen (O_2) consumption, enhanced glycolysis, depression of ATP consumption) enhanced glycolysis, depression of ATP consumption) with protective effects of endogenously released adenosine, with activates A1 receptors as well as certain types of K^+ channels (Kobayashi et al., 1995; Perez-Pinzon et al., 1997). These factors may also be responsible, in part, for the tolerance induced in hippocampal neurons by preconditioning motor activity. Such ischemic tolerance may depend on the reduction of nerve cell metabolism and energy demand. Ischemic preconditioning also facilitates the recovery of protein synthesis in CA1 after ischemia (Furuta et al., 1993; Nakagomi et al., 1993), proceeding in a lateral to medial direction, thereby mirroring the relative vulnerability (i.e. medial CA1>lateralCA1) of these neurons.

2.7. Mechanisms of Ischemic Tolerance in the Brain

Brain injury evolves over time, often taking days or even weeks to fully develop. It is a dynamic process that involves immediate oxidative stress and excitotoxicity followed by inflammation and preprogrammed cell death (Ferriero, 2005). Following focal ischemia, a complex and dynamic interaction of vascular cells, glial cells, and neurons determines the extent of the ensuing lesion (Trendelenburg et al., 2005). Traditionally, the focus has been on mechanisms of damage, while recently it has become clear that endogenous mechanisms of protection are equally important for the final outcome (Trendelenburg et al., 2005). Neuroprotective strategies include salvaging neurons through the use of targeted pharmacotherapies, protecting neurons through preconditioning, and repairing neurons by enhancing neurogenesis. Investigation of ischemic tolerance is mainly performed in different animal models. The precise mechanism of ischemic tolerance in the brain is yet not fully understood. However, numerous candidates exist as possible inductors, transductors and effectors of ischemic tolerance (see table 4). Some of these may contribute to delayed neuronal death, while others may protect against ischemia and facilitate cell survival. On the other side, it is generally accepted that systemic physiological parameters, such as changes of temperature or of CBF, have no direct influence on ischemic tolerance.

Table 4. Overview of rapid ischemic tolerance

Sensors:	ATP-sensitive K^+-channel
	Protein kinase C α/β
Transducer	adenosine
	adenosine receptor type
Effectors	ATP-sensitive K^+-channel

Legend. ATP: adenosine triphosphat.

There exist mainly 3 phases of ischemic tolerance: (*i*) induction, (*ii*) transduction and (*iii*) tolerance (Schaller et al., 2002). During *induction* phase, NMDA and adenosine receptors and, possibly, oxygen free radicals and conservation of energy metabolism are required. Protein kinases, transcription factors, and immediate early genes appear to transduce the signal into a tolerant response. Ischemic tolerance can be observed in at least two temporal profiles (see table 5): The *rapid phase of protection* lasts for several hours after the preconditioning stimulus. Adenosine receptors and ATP-sensitive potassium channels (K_{ATP}) may play a role similar to that in cardiac ischemic tolerance (Perez-Pinzon et al., 1997). The *delayed phase of protection*, retained for a maximum of 2-4 days, currently is best explained by de novo protein synthesis (Kitigawa et al., 1990). It has been hypothesized that the early and late windows of preconditioning may reflect changes in cellular metabolism and gene expression, respectively (Perez-Pinzon et al., 1997). Ischemic tolerance in the brain is usually of the delayed type, but in the heart, the tolerance induced by ischemic preconditioning is almost immediate and wanes quite rapidly within a few hours, representing a marked difference between the heart and the brain.

There is strong evidence that ischemic tolerance is a reproducible phenomenon, but its underlying mechanism is not entirely understood. A possible explanation of tolerance induction is the neuronal stress response. Although the stress response can be a major component of ischemic tolerance in the brain, neurons seem to be protected by divergent mechanisms of tolerance induction. Protein kinas signaling, immediate early genes, growth factors, and antioxidant defense enzymes are examples of such a response. It may not be surprising; therefore, that induction of ischemic tolerance is governed by multiple mechanisms.

In experimental models, complete or true neuroprotection can be achieved only through preconditioning, a process during which an animal develops tolerance to an otherwise lethal stressor. Although of no clinical use, preconditioning models have provided valuable insight into how repair systems work in the brain. Cumulative evidence indicates that the same genes that are up-regulated during preconditioning, those mediating true protection, are also up-regulated during injury and repair. Numerous mediators and mechanisms have been proposed to explain induced ischemic tolerance (Prass et al,. 2003). Specifically, hypoxic preconditioning and hypoxic-ischemic insult have been shown to induce hypoxia inducible factor-1 (HIF-1) and its target survival genes, vascular endothelial growth factor (VEGF), and erythropoietin (Epo) in rodents (Ferriero, 2005). Of particular interest is the up-regulation of Epo, a growth factor that may have therapeutic potential in the treatment of ischemic stroke (Schaller et al., 2006).

Table 5. Overview of rapid ischemic tolerance

Sensors	adenosine adenosine receptor type 1 oxygen free radical Hypoxia inducible factor NMDA receptor excitatory amino acid transporter 1-2 heme-containing sensor
Transducers	immediate-early gene/heat shock protein ATP-sensitive K+-channel extracellular signal-regulated kinase protein kinase B phosphoinositide-3-kinase C-jun N-terminal protein kinase nuclear-factor κB erythropoietin tumor necrosis factor ceramide nitric oxide synthase protein tyrosine phosphorylation protein kinase C $p21^{ras}$/extracellular signal-regulated kinase camp-response element
Effectors	mitogen-activated protein kinase heat-shock protein BCL proteins oxygen free radical scavenger brain-derived neutrotrophic factors vascular-endothelial growth factor downregulation of nitric oxide/nitric oxide synthase $GABA_A$ receptor upregulation IL-1-receptor antagonist Glutamate receptor subunit 2 downregulation

Legend: NMDA: N-methyl-D-aspartate, ATP: adenosine tri-phosphat; BCL: B-cell-lymphoma; GABA: gamma aminobutyric acid; IL-1: interleukin-1.

HIF-1 is a key physiological sensor of the oxygen level in most mammalian cells. Hypoxia induces HIF-1 p (Semenza, 2000), and HIF-1 then regulates the cellular transcriptional response to reduced oxygen availability to restore homeostasis of oxygen as a substrate for aerobic metabolism (Prass et al., 2003). In various models, activation of HIF-1 has been implicated as a key event in tolerance induction in vitro (Ruscher et al., 2002) and in vivo (Prass et al., 2003; Bergeron et al., 2000). Among others, HIF-1 induces Epo (Semenza, 2000). Only recently it was found that Epo is also expressed in the central nervous system and that it exerts potent neuroprotective effects (Ehrenreich, 2004). Epo transcription as well as

Epo translation has been found in preconditioned brains (Prass et al., 2002; Prass et al., 2003)). In addition, there is solid evidence that exogenously applied Epo is neuroprotective in vitro as well as in vivo (cited in Schaller et al., 2006). Epo may be necessary but not sufficient for neuroprotection (Schaller et al., 2006), so that it appears more likely that there are also other protective signaling cascades involved in hypoxia-induced tolerance in the brain that are independent of Epo (Prass et al., 2003; cited in Schaller et al., 2006). Potential candidates include NO, adenosine, vascular endothelial growth factor, Bcl-2, heat shock protein 70, and tumor necrosis factor-α.

The objective of ischemic preconditioning research is to identify the underlying endogenous protective cellular receptors and signaling cascades, with the long-term goal of allowing therapeutic augmentation of the endogenous protective mechanisms in cerebral ischemia and possibly development of new neuroprotective strategies for ischemic stroke treatment. At this time, however, the postinjury enhancement of neurogenesis appears to offer the best hope for long-lasting functional recovery following brain injury.

2.7.1. Ischemic Tolerance in the Heart

In the heart tissue, the main events suggested to occur in the process of acquisition of protection include initiation of the process by the release of several stress signal molecules (adenosine, bradykinin, opioids, endothelin and norepinephrine), stimulating receptors linked to activation of protein kinase C (PKC). The activation of PKC is followed by activation of other kinases, which carry the signal to mitochondrial K_{ATP}, followed by activation of transcription factors. The latter activate genes encoding various protective proteins, such as heat shock proteins and enzymes acting to neutralize reactive oxygen species (ROS) (Baxter, 2002). The above main events are interconnected by numerous mediators of the protection signal, suggested to include G proteins, phospholipase C-β1 (PLC-β1) and phospholipase D (PLD), diacylglycerol (DAG), nitric oxide, ROS, tyrosine kinases, mitogen-activated protein kinases (MAP-kinase), transcription factors and probably many other mediators (Nakano et al., 2000; Pagliaro et al., 2001; Schulz et al., 2001; Baxter, 2002).

2.7.2. Ischemic Tolerance in the Brain

As stated above, the elucidation of the ischemic preconditioning mechanism in the brain lags behind that in the heart. The brain was shown over a decade ago to possess the endogenous protective mechanism activated by ischemic preconditioning (Kitagawa et al., 1990; Kato et al., 1991; Kirino et al., 1991; Liu et al., 1992, 1993; Nishi et al., 1993; Kuzuya et al., 1993; Gidday et al., 1994; Kato et al., 1994a, 1994b).

Transient impairment of energy metabolism induces ischemic tolerance in the brain and ischemic tolerance is associated with improved preservation of energy metabolism and mitochondrial function (Schaller et al., 2002; Liu et al., 2002; Zhan et al., 2002) during the ischemic event. However, it is less clear whether ischemic tolerance affords protection by reducing energy expenditure (as in some anoxia-tolerant or hibernating animals), increasing high-energy phosphates, improving substrate delivery (e.g. increasing CBF or glucose transport), or improving the efficiency of energy metabolism (e.g. inducing glycolytic or respiratory-chain enzymes). Many ischemic tolerance mechanisms appear similar or identical to highly conserved responses to oxygen deprivation, in particular via the transcription factor HIF-1. HIF-1 sense hypoxia and transactives genes, leading to (among other things), vasculogenesis, increased glucose transport and increased gylcolysis. Not surprisingly, ischemic preconditioning can up-regulate activity of glucose-transporter-1 (GLUT-1) (Jones et al., 2001; Bernaudin et al., 2002), phosphofructokinase and lactate dehydrogenase (Jones et al., 2001).

Mechanisms, which are prominent during the excitotoxic phase of ischemic cell death (Dirnagl et al., 1999), can serve as targets of ischemic tolerance. Several ischemic mechanisms depend on glutamate-receptor and Ca^{2+} signaling. In many models, ischemic tolerance requires NMDA-receptor activation. Ischemic tolerance can affect the subunit composition of neurotransmitter receptors and can up-regulate inhibitory neurotransmitter. In particular, breakdown products of ATP (most importantly adenosine), the adenosine A1 receptor and ATP-sensitive $K^{+}(K_{ATP})$channels (Heurteaux et al., 1995) seem to play an important role in intercepting the early events of the cascade leading to ischemic cell death. Adenosine, the ischemia-induced degradation product of ATP, which was shown to participate in the activation of the protective myocardial mechanism, was also demonstrated to activate the protective brain mechanism (Goldberg et al., 1988; Krieglstein and Rischke, 1991; Rudolphi et al., 1992; Daval and Nicolas, 1994; Schubert et al.,1994; Reshef et al., 1996). Adenosine initiates the protective mechanism by activation of the adenosine A_1 (and probably also A_3) receptors on the cell outer membrane, prompting a cascade of cellular events assembling a protective signal transduction pathway leading to ischemic tolerance. Various models were developed in order to elucidate the adenosine-induced protective signal transduction pathway.

Lipopolysaccaride (LPS), the prototypic stimulus for expression of pro-inflammatory cytokines, can precondition brain against subsequent ischemia. Cytoprotection by LPS in the brain involves an increase in activity of superoxide dismutase and endothelial nitric oxide synthetase (Bordet et al., 2000). Interleukin-1 (IL-1) and tumor necrosis factor (TNF) are strongly up-regulated by PLS. Preconditioning with IL-1 protects CA1 hippocampal neurons form global ischemia in the gerbil, and an IL-1- receptor antagonist blocks this effect (Ohtsuki et al., 1996). Cytoprotective preconditioning with TNF induces manganese superoxide dismutase (MnSOD) (Wong et al., 1988). Preclinical stroke models and primary cultures of cortical neurons, cortical astrocytes and microvessel endothelial cells show that TNF and its downstream mediator ceramide are involved in tolerance signaling (Goodman et al., 1996; Nawashiro et al., 1997; Liu et al., 2000). Preconditioning with TNF and ceramide blocks recruitment of the Ca^{2+}-binding protein p300/CBP to the p65 nuclear-factor κB (NFκB)-binding site on DNA, which modifies NFκB gene expression, inhibits expression of pro-inflammatory intercellular-adhesion molecule 1 (ICAM-1) messenger ribonucleic acid (mRNA), and preserves expression of MnSOD.

2.7.3. Activation of Adenosine Receptors

Activation of the neuronal adenosine receptors by exposure of the neuronal cultures to adenosine, to the A_1 adenosine receptor agonist N6-(R)-phenylisopropyladenosine (R(-)-PIA), or to sub lethal ischemia, resulted in a significant protection against the ischemic and the combined ischemia/reperfusion insults (Reshef et al., 1996). 8-Sulphophenyl theophylline (SPT), a non-selective A_1/A_2 adenosine receptor antagonist (Armstrong et al., 1994), significantly decreased the protection effect induced by R(-)-PIA and by sub lethal exposure to IAA, proving the involvement of adenosine receptors in the acquisition of ischemic tolerance. The exposure of the neurons to R(-)-PIA, or to adenosine, resulted in a relatively long uninterrupted time-window of protection against the ischemia-reperfusion insult (Reshef et al., 1996). Probably, this time-window of protection reflects a combination of the two separated time-windows of protection reported in the heart and in some brain models (early-immediate window lasting for hours and late-delayed window lasting for days). Indeed, in the experimental model of group around Zoref-Shani the time response curves for the protection effect induced by adenosine and R(-)-PIA against the ischemia/reperfusion insult, are compatible with two peaks of protection, one at 3 hour and the second at 48 hours (see for example Reshef et al., 1996).

2.7.4. Activation of Phospholipase C

Adenosine receptors are G-protein coupled receptors (GPCR). Therefore they could be anticipated to mediate the protection signal downstream to PLC (probably PLC-β1) through G-proteins (Fredholm et al., 2000; Freund et al., 1994; Munshi et al.,1991; Rhee et al., 1997; Schulte and Fredholm, 2003). Indeed, PLC was demonstrated to be activated in myocardial cultures by an agonist of the adenosine A_1 receptor (Parsons et al., 2000). The involvement of PLC in the neuronal adenosine- activated STP was demonstrated very recently (Rogel et al., 2004) by the findings that the PLC inhibitor U73122 abolished the R(-)-PIA -induced protection (see Figure 6) and that exposure of the neuronal cultures to R(-)-PIA resulted in activation of PLC (see Figure 7).

2.7.5. Activation of Proteinkinase C

Exposure of the cultures to the PKC activators 1,2 dioctanoyl-rac-glycerol (DOG) or phorbol 12-myristate 13-acetate (PMA) conferred a wide time-window of protection against the ischemic and ischemia/reperfusion insults, appearing immediately and extending up to 2 to 6 days, depending on the PKC modulating substance, the type of insult and the method of assessment of cell injury (Reshef et al., 1997). PKC is a family of some 11 serine/threonine specific protein kinase isozymes, which by phosphorylation of various cellular proteins, affect many cellular functions (Nishizuka, 1986; Huang et al., 1988; Nishizuka, 1989).

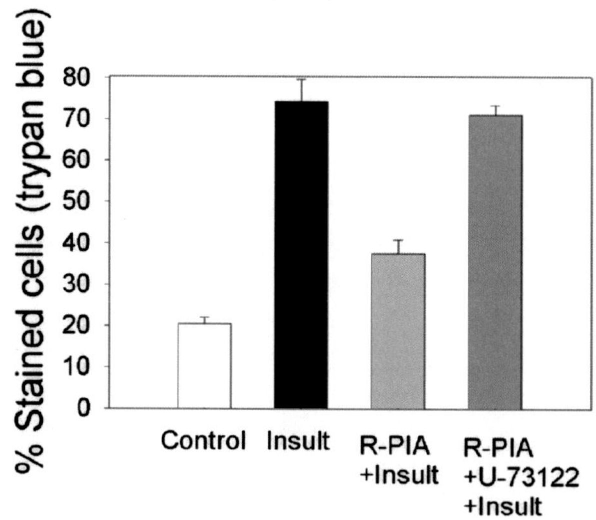

Figure 6. Abrogation of the R-PIA-induced protection by the PLC inhibitor U73122 (with permission of E. Zoref-Shani, Israel). Neuronal cultures were subjected to the experimental protocol as described in the Methods. Each bar represents mean ± SEM for 3 experiments, each performed in triplicates. P for the attenuation effect (protection) by R(-)-PIA of cell injury, in comparison to the non protected control was 0.001; Exposure of the cultures to U73122 abolished the protection induced by R(-)-PIA (the injury in presence of this inhibitor did not differ significantly from that in the non protected control, but differed significantly from the injury in the R-PIA-treated cells, $P<0.001$).

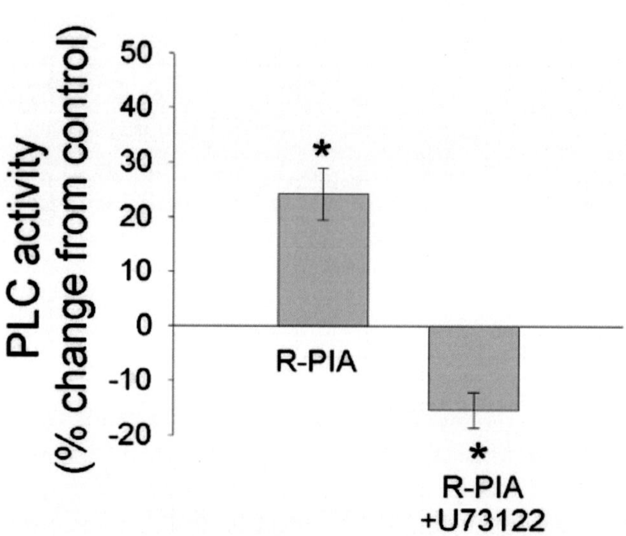

Figure 7. R-PIA enhances PLC activity (with permission of E. Zoref-Shani, Israel). Neuronal cultures prelabeled with $[^3H]$inositol, as described by Parsons et al., [Parsons et al., 2000], were incubated with R(-)-PIA (1 μM) for 30 min. Other cultures were incubated with U73122 (10 μM) for 10 min before the addition of R-PIA. Control cultures were incubated with DMSO (vehicle for R-PIA and U73122). Following incubation, the products of PLC activity were quantified [Parsons et al., 2000]. Results represent mean ± SEM of 4 to 10 experiments, each performed in triplicates. $*P<0.001$.

Modulation of PKC activity may be part of both protective and destructive signal transduction pathways, by decreasing or increasing intracellular calcium concentration, respectively (Iwasa and Hosey, 1984; Swartz, 1993). Some of the PKC isoforms mediate protective mechanisms, whereas others mediate destructive mechanisms, activated by different signals (Miettinen et al., 1996; Goodal et al., 1997; Buchner et al., 1999). Further proof for the participation of PKC activation in the R(-)-PIA-induced signal transduction pathway was obtained by demonstrating that bisindolylmaleimide I, a highly selective PKC inhibitor (Toullec et al., 1991), abolished the R(-)-PIA-induced protection (Di Capua et al., 2003). Additional studies disclosed conclusively the identity of the protecting PKC isoform to be PKC-ε (Di Capua et al., 2003). This identification was based on the following findings: Exposure of the cultures to R(-)-PIA resulted in phosphorylation (activation) of PKC-ε, but not of two other isoforms studied (α and δ). The increase in the amount of phosphorylated PKC-ε was observed immediately following the short exposure to R(-)-PIA and lasted for at least 6 hours. This finding may be taken to suggest that a long lasting dwelling of activated PKC-ε in its active state may be part of the "memory" mechanism, enabling the neurons to maintain the protective capacity for days. A more conclusive evidence that PKC-ε is the mediator of the protection signal was further obtained by demonstrating that insertion into the cells of εV1-2, a specific PKC-ε translocation inhibitor peptide (Johnson et al., 1996) (but not of εV1-2-s, the scrambled version of the inhibitor peptide (Yedovitzky et al., 1997), abrogated the protection conferred by R(-)-PIA (Di Capua et al., 2003). These findings provided, for the first time, conclusive evidence that PKC-ε mediates the protection signal against ischemia/reperfusion in the neuronal adenosine-activated signal transduction pathway. Moreover, this role of PKC-ε appears to be mandatory for the pathway, since blockage of PKC-ε activation abolished the protection.

It was not as yet identify the destructive PKC isoform, presumably activated in the neurons by ischemia/reperfusion or by other stresses. In isolated perfused rat hearts, PKC-δ was demonstrated to mediate the destructive signal, whereas activation of PKC-ε was found to mimic ischemic preconditioning (Inagaki et al., 2003).

2.7.6. Opening of K_{ATP} Channels

In the heart, the role of opening of the K_{ATP} channels in the acquisition of ischemic tolerance by the ischemic preconditioning mechanism was demonstrated in numerous studies (Cole, 1993; Rohmann et al., 1994; Bernardo et al., 1999; Fryer et al., 1999; Oldenburg et al., 2002). A similar role for opening of the K_{ATP} channels was established also in the brain (Murphy and Greenfield, 1991; Heurteaux et al., 1993; Haddad and Jiang, 1994; Heurteaux et al., 1995; Lauritzen et al., 1997). In the experimental model of Zoref-Shani, the protective role of opening of the channels was confirmed by demonstrating that glibenclamide (a channel blocker) abolished the protection induced by sub lethal ischemia and by the adenosine A_1 receptor agonist R(-)-PIA, as well as the protection conferred by DOG, throughout the entire time window of protection induced by these substances (Reshef et al., 1998; 2000b). The induction of protection through opening of the K_{ATP} channels by DOG, is in accordance with the knowledge that opening of the K_{ATP} channels during ischemia, depends on their prior phosphorylation (priming) by activated PKC (Ashcroft, 1988; Cole, 1993; Edwards and Weston, 1993; Wann, 1993; Haddad and Jiang, 1994; Grover, 1996; Light et al., 1996; Liu et al., 1996). The finding that glibenclamide abolished completely the protection induced by R(-)-PIA and by DOG, throughout the entire time window of protection induced by these substances, may be taken to suggest that prolonged state of activation of these channels underlies the long memory of the protection capacity. It could also reflect the combined operation of several different adenosine-induced protective mechanisms, all depending on opening of the K_{ATP} channels, but each maturating at a different time point. Prolonged state of activated channels may also reflect long half-life of activated PKC-ε, priming the channels continuously.

The mechanism by which opening of the K_{ATP} channels confers ischemic tolerance is not yet completely clarified (Garlid et al., 2003). One possible mechanism may be associated with preservation of ATP. Opening of the membranal K_{ATP} channels in the neurons results in repolarization or hyperpolarization, reducing membrane excitability, down-regulating neuronal metabolic and energy consuming activity (Wann, 1993). Another K_{ATP} channels-dependent protective mechanism may be associated with generation of ROS (Garlid et al., 2003). Moderate generation of ROS was implicated in the preconditioning mechanism (Das et al., 1999; Ravati et al., 2000, 2001) and opening of the channels was demonstrated to cause moderate bursts of ROS release (Pain et al., 2000; Forbes et al., 2001; Garlid et al., 2003). The generated ROS may activate kinases which mediate the protective signal, or participate in post translational modification of proteins to become protective (Baxter, 2002). A mitochondrial K_{ATP} channels signal amplification loop was suggested to operate in the heart (Garlid et al., 2003). According to this suggestion, the ROS generated during opening of the channels by ischemic preconditioning (a step occurring probably downstream to the activation of PKC), activate kinases that are probably upstream to PKC (see figure 3). The proposed end result of the loop is to phosphorylate the channels, putting it in a long-lived open state (Garlid et al., 2003).

2.8. Hypothesized Adenosine-Induced Signal Transduction Pathway (Suggested by Zoref-Shani)

In view of experimental studies, performed in the brain and heart, Zoref-Sahni and her Israeli group suggest a hypothesized scheme for the cascade of events leading in the neurons from activation of the adenosine receptors to the acquisition of ischemic tolerance (see Figure 8). Adenosine receptors are GPCR, known to mediate signals down stream, through G-proteins, to PLC-β1 and probably also through PLD. They demonstrated recently the involvement of PLC in the R(-)-PIA-induced protection (Rogel et al., 2004). PLC catalyzes the synthesis of diacylglycerol (DAG), which is associated with activation of PKC. The activated PKC-ε primes (phosphorylates) the K_{ATP} channels, resulting in opening of the channels during a subsequent energy crisis (increased adenosine diphosphate (ADP)/ATP ratio). Opening of the channels is an obligatory event for the acquisition of the whole (relatively long) duration of protection. However, the cascade of events leading from opening of the channels to this protection is not yet completely clarified (Garlid et al., 2003). The mechanism by which opening of the channels confers the immediate protection is especially unclear. It could reflect the effect of channel opening to diminish ATP consumption (Wann, 1993). The mechanism leading to the delayed protection is hypothesized to be associated with release of moderate bursts of ROS from the opened channels (Pain et al., 2000; Forbes et al., 2001; Garlid et al., 2003) (see figure 3). The role of ROS in damaging cells is well established (Droge, 2002). Nevertheless, moderate generation of ROS was implicated in many normal physiological processes in the cells (Droge, 2002). Indeed, moderate generation of ROS was implicated in the preconditioning mechanism in the heart, through activation of various kinases (Das et al., 1999; Ravati et al., 2000, 2001; Baxter, 2002; Garlid et al., 2003). The ROS-activated kinases were suggested to mediate the protective signal to transcription factors, activating genes encoding protective proteins. ROS-activated kinases may also participate in post translational modulation of the protective proteins produced as a result of activation of the transcription factors (Baxter, 2002). As a representative of the non receptor tyrosine kinases, we chose to clarify first if the family of v-src sarcoma (Schmidt-Ruppin A-2) viral oncogene homologue (avian) (Src) tyrosine kinases participates in the adenosine-activated mechanism and whether its activation is associated with PKC-ε. This choice was made in view of the following data. Protein tyrosine kinases were demonstrated in recent years to be involved in various preconditioning signaling pathways in the heart (Vahlhause et al.,1998; Dawn et al., 1999; Fryer et al., 1999; Dana et al., 2000; Cohen et al., 2000; Okubo et al., 2000; Ping et al., 2002). Src-protein kinases, a specific subgroup family of protein tyrosine kinases (Brown and Cooper 1996; Sicheri and Kuriyan 1997; Bjorge et al., 2000; Ma and Huang, 2002), were demonstrated to be involved in myocardial preconditioning signaling (Ping et al., 1999; Hattori et al., 2001; Vondriska et al., 2001; Dawn and Bolli 2002; Dawn et al., 2002b; Qin et al., 2002), as well as in neuronal nicotinic receptor-mediated protection against glutamate and β-amyloid-induced neurotoxicity (Kihara et al., 2001).

Among the transcription factors we suspect the participation of NFkB. Like the case of ROS (see above), also NFkB can operate in both destructive and protective pathways (Shou et al,. 2002; Chiarugi, 2002; Kukreja, 2002; Baxter, 2002). NFkB is a well characterized apoptosis signal (for example, causing up-regulation of Bcl-X_S, Bax and release of cytochrome C from mitochondria (Shou et al, 2002), but there are reports that NFkB may also be involved in the mediation of protective signals, such as the myocardial delayed protection signal. Activation of NFkB can result in activation of protective genes, encoding the synthesis of NFkB–dependent antiapoptotic proteins, such as Bcl-x_L, Bcl-2 and A1/Bfl-1, cIAP-2, A20, heat shock proteins of the 70 kDa family and the antioxidant enzyme MnSOD (Chiarugi et al. 2002; Kukreja et al., 2002; Baxter et al., 2002). An additional possibility of conferring protection through modulation of NFkB activation, is that the adenosine-induced protection signal inhibits the NFkB-dependent apoptosis signal. The mechanism directing NFkB translocation to the nucleus to activation of proapoptotic or antiapoptotic genes, is of major interest in contemporary molecular biology (Perkins et al., 2000; Kukreja et al., 2002).

Our knowledge concerning the adenosine-induced signal transduction pathway, which confers protection to neurons against ischemia-reperfusion insult, was enhanced considerably during the last decade. Yet, much is still to be learned on this mechanism in order to completely unravel the phenomenon.

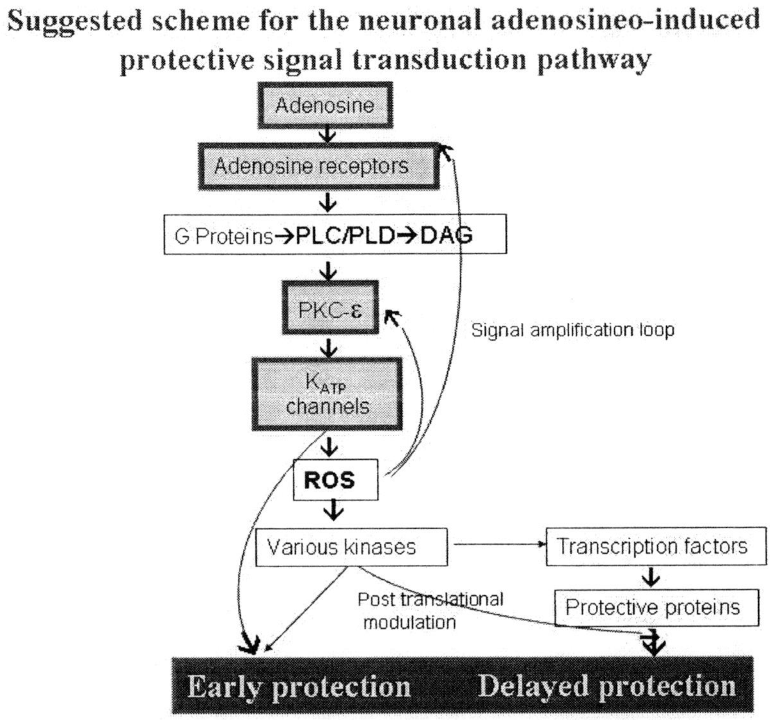

Legend: PLC: phospholipase C; PLD: phospholipase D; DAG: diacylglycerol; PKC: proteinkinase C; K_{ATP}: ATP-sensitive K^{+}channels; ROS: reactive oxygen species. See text fordetailed explanations.

Figure 8. Proposed schematic diagram of the neuronal adenosine-induced signal transduction pathway leading to ischemic tolerance. (with permission of E. Zoref-Shani, Israel).

2.9. Ischemic Tolerance and Postischemic Functional Recovery

It has been postulated that neuronal protection by ischemic tolerance is only a transient phenomenon. After acquisition of ischemic tolerance, Corbett and Crooks (Corbett et al., 1997) recognized a gradual decline of CA1 neurons that were initially protected from ischemia. They observed that neuronal loss continued in the CA1 sector with increasing survival time. The decrease depended on the age of the animals. In older animals, the decline in neuronal number was slow and mild, whereas young gerbils showed a faster and greater decrease in number. Ischemic tolerance protected around 85% of CA1 neurons in old and young gerbils. The number decreased down to 53-65% in young animals at 60 days protection, but it did not on the second day after drug administration (Ohtsuki et al., 1992). Keeping in mind that experimental work of ischemic flow threshold has demonstrated the existence of 2 critical levels of decreased perfusion: (*i*) a level below which reversible neuronal failure occurs (functional threshold) and (*ii*) a lower threshold below which irreversible membrane failure and morphological damage occurs (Heiss, 1992), these experimental data demonstrate a gradual development of neuronal functional recovery.

Brain resistance to ischemic injury is not limited to ischemic ischemic preconditioning but has also been observed after other tissue stresses such as heat shock treatment (Kitagawa et al., 1991) and chemical metabolic stress (Riepe et al., 1997). In addition, ischemic tolerance can be produced by spreading depression (a common ischemia-related phenomenon). Indeed, spreading depression can induce ischemic tolerance (Kobayashi et al., 1995, Matsushima et al., 1996), and this appears to activate glial cells (Kraig et al., 1991), suggesting that increased support by these cells may be involved in subsequent neuroprotection. Available data suggest that threshold depolarizations required to induce tolerance are comparable to those that induce transcription factor mRNAs (e.g., c-*fos*), while that inducing heat shock protein 72 (Hsp72) approaches closer to the threshold for neuronal injury (Kobayashi et al., 1995; Abe et al., 1996). The coordinated expression of protective antioxidant enzymes (Toyoda et al., 1997) and nerve growth factors (Hsu et al., 1993; Takeda et al., 1993) may also be involved in ischemic tolerance. In addition, ischemic preconditioning might alter tissue metabolism in a manner that sustains ischemic tolerance tissue by providing an increased penumbra and a reduced ischemic core zone, without altering blood flow. Finally, ischemic preconditioning might attenuate later postischemic leukocyte adhesion and emigration (Akimitsu et al., 1996).

2.10. Necrosis, Apoptosis and Ischemic Tolerance – The Same Pathway?

It may be hypothesized that the initial steps in the pathways of neuronal apoptosis, and necrosis may be similar with regards to participating mediators. The intensity of the stimulus may be of great importance in the way, that a maximal stimulation of NMDA receptors leads to necrosis (Eguchi et al., 1997) and a submaximal stimulation to apoptosis (Eugchi et al., 1997). Such assumption is supported by in vitro data showing that apoptotic degeneration occurs at 43-45°C and necrotic degeneration at >45°C (Lennon et al., 1991). Interestingly, the question as to whether a cell will degenerate through apoptotic or necrotic pathways, depends not only on strength and duration of harmful stimuli but also on intracellular ATP levels (Leist et al., 1997). One may assume in this concept, that a median stimulation of NMDA receptors induces, as a third pathway, programmed cell protection (delayed preconditioning).

Ischemia induces genes that regulate apoptosis, including bax (found in cells destined to die) and bcl-2 (found in cells that survive) (Graham et al., 2002). In some ischemic tolerance models, bcl-2 protein induction parallels initiation and cessation of tolerance, and bcl-2 antisense oligonucleotides block tolerance (Shimizu et al., 2001). The transcription factors driving the induction of bcl-2 during tolerance include the camp-response-element-binding protein (CREB), as the bcl-2 promoter contains a camp-response element (CRE). Multiple protein kinases can activate transcription via the CRE, by phosphorylation of CREB (Walton et al., 2000). Presumably, blc-2 acts at the mitochondria, where the up-regulation of base excision repair capability distinguished tolerance from ischemic damage (Chen et al. 2003). Protein-synthesis-dependent tolerance to ischemia occurs in the absence of bcl-2 induction, supporting the idea that there are multiple effectors (Wick et al., 2002).

2.11. Stress Proteins and Ischemic Tolerance

Acquisition of ischemic tolerance could be explained by the stress response of the brain (see table 6). When exposed to a noxious environment, the stress signal in the cell is transferred to heat-shock factors to convey information to the heat-shock element that exist upstream to stress-inducible hsp genes. Then, hsp gene expression is greatly enhanced and the cell acquires transient tolerance to further stresses. These characteristics are common to a wide variety of cells, and neurons may not be the exception. The stress response is essential for cell survival because cells cannot cope with a sudden accumulation of denatured proteins or protein aggregation that arise from various stresses such as thermal, anoxic or oxidative stresses. Protein aggregates do not accumulate in unstressed cells because they are continuously degraded by cellular health control machinery. This mechanism consists of chaperoning unfolded proteins and subsequent proteolysis by the ubiquitin-proteasome pathway (Chiechanover et al., 2000). Approximately one third of newly synthesized proteins, in fact, are degraded within minutes of their synthesis (Yewdell et al., 2001).

When ischemic tolerance is induced by preceding ischmia, Hsp70 increases in the hippocampal CA1 pyramidal cell in the gerbil (Liu et al., 1993) and in the rat (Galzier et al., 1994). The amount of Hsp70 was also shown to correlate well with tolerance acquisition in a gerbil model of chronic hypoperfusion of the brain (Ohtsuki et al., 1993). Increased amounts of Hsp70 seem to be necessary for ischemic tolerance, since experimental manipulation that inhibits Hsp70 function abolishes ischemic tolerance (Nakata et al., 1993). Other stress proteins were also reported to increase on tolerance induction. An increase of Hsp27 was demonstrated in the brain after tolerance (Kato et al., 1992). The direct role of Hsp27 in neuronal ischemic tolerance remains to be explained since Hsp27 expression is observed mainly in glial cells. Induction of the Hsp110/105 family was studied in rats that had acquired ischemic tolerance by transient ischemia (Yagita et al., 2001). Colocalization of Hsp110/105 and hsp70 in the CA1 neurons suggested that expression of these stress proteins contribute to ischemic tolerance.

Table 6. Stress proteins

Family	Name	Location
Hsp100	Hsp100	cytosol
Hsp90	Hsp90	cytosol
	Grp94	endoplasmatic reticulum
Hsp70	Hsc70 (HspA8)	cytosol
	Hsp70	cytosol
	BiP	endoplasmatic reticulum
Hsp60	Hsp60	mitochondria
SmallHsp	Hsp27	
	aA and aB-crystallin ubiquitin	

Legend: Hsp:heat shock protein.

It is well established that protein synthesis is impaired by cerebral ischemia (Kleihues et al., 1971). When ischemic tolerance was induced in the gerbil model, the recovery phase of protein synthesis was accelerated after ischemia (Furuta et al., 1993). Autoradiography using isotope-labeled amino acids demonstrated a good recovery, and the pattern of amino acid incorporation in the CA1 neurons returned to a normal pattern within 24 hours. Ultrastructural distribution of aggregated ribosomes was also restored to a near-normal pattern within 24 hours (Furuta et al., 1993). Autoradiography using isotope-labeled amino acids demonstrated a good recovery, and the pattern of amino acid incorporation in the CA1 neurons returned to a normal pattern within 24 hours. Ultrastructural distribution of aggregated ribosomes was also restored to a near-normal pattern within 24 hours (Furuta et al., 1993). Stress-inducible proteins such as ubiquitin and Hsp70 do not appear after 5 minutes of ischemia in the gerbil model. After 2 minutes of ischemia that induces ischemic tolerance, however, expression of ubiquitin (Furuta et al., 1993) and Hsp70 (Aoki et al., 1993) is enhanced. Ischemic tolerance also facilitated recovery of the synthesis of superoxide dismutase and, presumably, thereby protected neurons from ischemia (Toyoda et al., 1997). These experimental results have shown that ischemia disrupts the protein-synthesizing machinery, but ischemic tolerance can accelerate its recovery.

2.12. Cross Tolerance

Cross-tolerance implies that a noxious stress can confer cellular tolerance to a subsequent stress that is different in nature from the first one (see table 7). In different animal models, it has been demonstrated that ischemic preconditioning could be induced by different metabolic, pharmacological, inflammatory and physical stimulations.

In general, the ischemic tolerance phenomenon exists for several days in-vivo experiment using rodents and thus, such time window of protective effect may have a limitation of clinical utility. Cross tolerance facilitates the induction of the pathophysiological cascade that has been reported to be demonstrating cytoprotective effects in vivo. This induction of ischemic cross-tolerance can be viewed from the perspective of when they are administered. Intraischemic and postischemic interventions have been demonstrated to be effective in limiting ischemic brain damage. One of the draw-backs of most preconditioning stimuli is that they are also capable of producing brain tissue damage with only minor changes in their intensity or duration. In the case of ischemia-induced ischemic tolerance, the safety margin in extremely narrow. Although other preconditioning stimuli than ischemic do not all require invasive procedures in experimental settings, these inductions have inherent dangers (e.g. toxicity) that could preclude their use in the clinical setting. Nonetheless, the need for an effective means of treating anticipated periods of ischemia remains acute, and continuous to stimulate the evaluation of a variety of conditioning stimuli. The ideal goal of these efforts is to identify an effective, non-invasive form of preconditioning that possesses an acceptable safety margin.

Stresses such as status epilepticus and hypoglycemia are also inducers of the stress response and can bring about ischemic tolerance. In contrast, hypothermia that usually suppress the stress response was shown to reduce subsequent cerebral infarction.

Table 7. Inducers of ischemic tolerance

Inducers of ischemic tolerance	Inducers of cross-tolerance
Sublethal global (forebrain) ischemia	hyperthermia (heat stress)
Brief transient focal ischemia	anoxia/hypoxia
	spreading depression
	epilepsy
	inhibition of oxidative phosphorylation (3-nitropropionate)
	oxidative stress (diethyldithiocarbamate)
	lipopolysaccaride
	traumatic brain injury
	hypothermia

2.13. Different Experimental Induction of Ischemic Tolerance

2.13.1. Pharmacological preconditioning

Preconditioning can be initiated also pharmacologically that is by drugs administered before the ischemic event, with an intervening washout period before the ischemic event (true pharmacological preconditioning) or without a washout period (more appropriately called a pharmacological pretreatment). Among others, preconditioning can be triggered by substances like (*i*) adenosine, (*ii*) bradykinin, (*iii*) NO, (*iv*) the mitochondrial K_{ATP}-channel opener diazoxide, (*v*) PKC activators, (*vi*) opioids, and also (*vii*) prostaglandins (for review see Post et al., 2002).

2.13.2. Thrombin Preconditioning

Decreased CBF during hibernating is accompanied by neuroprotective adaptations to this „low-flow“ state, such as reduced members of circulating leukocytes and platelets as well as increased clotting time. Such changes likely offer protection by suppressing thrombus formation.

Low concentration of thrombin is neuroprotective in vitro and in vivo. In vitro studies have shown that thrombin protects rat primary astrocytes from hypoglycemia or oxidative stress induced cell death. Thrombin also protects rat primary hippocampal neurons from cell death produced by hypoglycemia, hypoxia or growth supplements deprivation (Striggow et al., 2000). In addition, thrombin attenuates neuronal cell death and modulates astrocyte reactivity induced by β-amyloid in vitro. The effect of thrombin on both neurons and astrocytes is mimicked by thrombin receptor-activating peptide and inhibited by two potent thrombin inhibitors, hirudin and protease nexin-1 (Pike et al., 1996). Furthermore, thrombin pretreatment prevents cell damage induced by a large dose of thrombin in vitro (Jinag et al.,

2002). In vivo studies have demonstrated that intracerebral infusion of a low dose of thrombin reduces the brain damage that follows a subsequent intracerebral infusion of a high dose of thrombin, an intracerebral hemorrhage or cerebral ischemia (Xi et al., 2000). Thrombin pretreatment significantly attenuated the brain edema, which normally follows the infusion of a large dose of thrombin. This effect was abolished by a thrombin inhibitor, hirudin (Xi et al., 1999). Thrombin preconditioning may also be an important component of ischemic tolerance as the thrombin inhibitor, hirudin, can block ischemic tolerance in the brain (Jiang et al., 2002). Although the precise mechanism of thrombin-induced ischemic tolerance is not known, activation of thrombin receptors, up-regulation of thrombin inhibitors and heat shock proteins in the brain may be associated with the induced tolerance (Jiang et al., 2002). The majority of cellular functions influenced by thrombin are mediated by thrombin receptors (poly(ADP-ribosylation (PAR)-1, -3, and –4) under physiological conditions (Coughlin, 2000). Thrombin receptor activation is involved in the protection induced by thrombin preconditioning as the effect is mimicked by a thrombin receptor agonist and suppressed by a thrombin receptor antagonist both in vivo and in vitro (Jiang et al., 2002). Activation of thrombin receptor is associated with neuroprotection induced by thrombin (Jiang et al., 2002). Prior activation of thrombin receptor by either thrombin receptor-activating peptide or by thrombin resulted in full protection of thrombin receptor mRNA levels under hypoxic condition (Landau et al., 2000). Endogenous thrombin inhibitors such as plasminogen activator inhibitor-1 (PAI-1) may be responsible for thrombin-induced brain protection. PAI-1 content is increased after intracerebral infusion of thrombin in a dose-dependent manner, as well as after intracerebral hemorrhage and cerebral ischemia. Hirudin blocks the up-regulation of PAI-1 after intracerebral hemorrhage indicating a role for thrombin (Hua et al., 2000). PAI-1 appears to be neuroprotective as it reduces NMDA-induced neurotoxicity (Buisson et al,. 1998) and ischemic infarct volume is increased in PAI-1 knockout mice (Nagai et al., 1999). However, the protective effect conferred by PAI-1 may not be a result of its action against thrombin alone because PAI-1 is also an inhibitor of recombinant tissue plasminogen activator (tPA).

2.13.3. Erythropoetin Preconditioning

Astrocytes are the main cellular source of the glcoyprotein hormone epo in the brain, and low oxygen tension stimulates epo-mRNA expression in astrocytes (Ruscher et al., 2002). Besides astrocytes, epo receptors have been detected in neurons as well (Ruscher et al., 2002). Epo has been suggested as another endogenous mediator of preconditioning induced tolerance since it is produced in the brain tissue after ischemic stroke (Digicaylioglu et al., 2001; Heiss et al., 1999). Epo acts as a transducer in a signaling cascade in which HIF-1α is the sensor. Epo induces a phosphorylation cascade, including the Janus kinase-2 pathway, the phosphoinositide-3 kinase (Ruscher et al., 2002) or Akt (Siren et al., 2001) pathway, and the extracellular signaling-regulated kinase (ERK) and signal transducers or activators of the transcription pathway (Digicaylioglu et al., 2001), which converges on effectors of the bcl-protein family to protect neurons from apoptosis.

Although epo is suggested to present a major role in ischemic preconditioning (Dawson, 2002), this function has not been proven, nor has it yet been demonstrated that it is directly induced by ischemic preconditioning. Indeed, neuronal expression of epo is shown to be reduced after stimuli that induce ischemic preconditioning (Jones et al., 2001): lethal stimuli, especially hypoxic ischemia, clearly induce epo, but it seems that sublethal preconditioning stimuli are not potent enough to induce substantial concentrations of epo (Jones et al., 2001). Despite the lack of direct evidence that epo mediates ischemic preconditioning, epo may be an ideal exogenous preconditioning agent. A more definitive proof for a functional role of epo in preconditioning has been provided by previous studies demonstrating that the exogenous application of serum erythropoietin receptor (sEPOR) as an inhibitor of endogenous epo, attenuates the protective effect of oxygen-glucose deprivation in an in vitro model of stroke (Pfenninger et al., 1997), or hypoxia in a focal animal model of stroke (Ruscher et al., 2002). In case of protection of peritumoral tissue, there exist only a few preliminary data. A caveat to the use of epo as a neurotherapeutic modality is the potentially deleterious expansion of the red cell mass (hematocrit) and increased platelet aggregability. Asioloepo, a deglycoxylated congener of epo, crosses the blood brain barrier (BBB) and provides neuroprotection, but does not significantly affect the hematocrit (Ruscher et al,. 2002). Further experiments will be required to determine whether asialoepo preconditioning recapitulates the glioprotective effects. In addition, it seems that epo may enhance neurogenesis in both neonatal and adult animals following ischemia (Ferriero, 2005).

In a proof-of-principle trial, epo demonstrated a significant effect in stroke patients in both clinical outcome and recovery of infarcted brain tissue (Ehrenreich, 2004). Thus, epo stands out from different neuroprotective treatment options that have failed to be successfully transferred from animal models to human patients (Ehrenreich, 2004; Ehrenreich et al., 2002).

2.13.4. Hyopthermia Preconditioning

Hypothermia is capable to induce ischemic tolerance. This phenomenon is initiated under these conditions within 6 hours of preconditioning, persists for at least two days, and is completed by 7 days. The time course over which hypothermia-induced tolerance occurs, and the ability of aniosmycin to block tolerance, suggest that increased expression of one or more gene products underlies as mechanism to this phenomenon. Evidence suggests that delayed tolerance induced by hypothermic preconditioning is also due to direct cellular changes in the brain parenchyma. Synaptic responses showed significantly better posthypoxic recovery in slices prepared from preconditioned animals than in slices from non-preconditioned animals. Inasmuch as systemic variables, such a CBF and temperature, do not play a role in the slice neurons and/or glia. It is important to stress that these findings do not rule a neuroprotective effect resulting from changes in systemic variables in the in vivo setting; CBF alterations could occur, in addition to direct changes in neurons and glia. However, these findings indicate that one or more cell types in the brain parenchyma become tolerant.

The value of hypothermic preconditioning in the clinical setting clearly remains to be established. Experimental findings indicate that clinical evaluation of hypothermic preconditioning may be warranted. Hypothermia exhibits several desirable features of a candidate mechanism for inducing tolerance. First, hypothermia is a noninvasive treatment. Second, although not without side effects, hypothermia exhibits a substantial safety margin with respect to neuronal injury (Chopp et al., 1992). Third, hypothermia-induced tolerance is expressed, and declines, over a manageable time course (Schaller et al., 2003). Inasmuch as hypothermia is already an approved clinical procedure for intraischemic and postischemic therapy, it is possible that hypothermia could provide a clinically useful conditioning stimulus for limiting injury elicited by anticipated periods of ischemia.

2.13.5. Other Substances

Glutamate has long been known to damage neurons by NMDA receptor-mediated mechanism. Paradoxically, subtoxic concentration of NMDA protect neurons against glutamate-mediated excitotoxicity (Jiang et al., 2003). One of the major mechanism of NMDA neurprotection involves the activation of NMDA receptors leading to the rapid release of brain derived neurotrophic factor (BDNF). BDNF then binds to and activates its cognate receptor, receptor tyrosine kinase B. The efficient utilization of these two receptors types confers remarkable resistance against millimolar concentrations of glutamate that damage more than 80% of neurons in the absence of preconditioning the neurons with a subtoxic concentration of NMDA. Exactly how the neurons mediate neuroprotection by activation of both receptors is just beginning to be understood. Both NMDA and tyrosine kinase B receptors activate nuclear factor κB (NF-κB), a transcription factor known to be involved in protecting neurons against many different kinds of toxic-induced ischemia. By converging on survival transcription factors, such as NF-κB, NMDA and tyrosine kinase receptor B receptors protect neurons (Jiang et al., 2003). Thus, crosstalk between these very different receptors provides a rapid means of neuronal communication to up-regulate survival proteins through release and transcriptional activation of mRNA.

2.14. From Animal Experiments to Clinical Practice

As our knowledge of cerebral ischemic preconditioning is almost limited to animal or in vitro models, a transfer of these results to the clinical daily routine is yet not possible. In animal models of global and focal ischemia neuroprotection is typically determined by quantifying the degree of cell loss or reduction in infarct volume shortly after the ischemic event. These methods are unable to reliably detect more subtle forms of neuronal death and dysfunction that arise from damage to non-homogenous cell populations (e.g. hilar and striatal neurons), or to dentrides (e.g. loss of structural proteins or decreased synaptic transmission). It is argued that this type of covert damage contributes to a wide range of functional impairments (e.g. decreased working memory, altered filed potentials, loss of forelimb dexterity) that are rarely used as outcome measures in experimental studies even though they are of paramount importance clinically. The therapeutic window for certain treatment options is not necessarily the same either (STAIR, 1999).

One of the main conditions that an experimental model must meet is to reproduce the clinical situation as far as possible, but the experimental situation itself established differences that can contribute to the lack of agreement between laboratory results and clinical studies. One of these differences is due to the homogeneity intended in the laboratory, as regards parameters with a potential influence, to facilitate the achievement of valid conclusions. This homogeneity is far from being achieved in clinical conditions: patients have arterial occlusions at different sites, and the efficacy of collateral circulation changes from one patient to another, as do the physiological parameters.

2.15. Clinical Aspects of Cerebral Ischemic Tolerance

Ischemic tolerance has attracted little attention in clinical stroke research. However, apart from the above-mentioned problems to transfer the experimental data to the clinical practice, there is already clinical evidence to support the phenomenon of ischemic tolerance in the human brain.

2.15.1. Prestroke Transient Ischemic Attack

The first description of this ischemic tolerance-phenomenon was in the heart, which was reported by Murry in 1986 (Murry et al., 1986). Subsequent studies demonstrated ischemic preconditioning in lung, kidney and liver tissue, whereas more recent studies have concentrated on the brain during the years after.

TIA have long been identified as a risk factor for subsequent ischemic stroke. However, recent clinical evidence suggests that prestroke TIA may improve neurological outcome after stroke (Moncayo et al., 2000; Weih et al., 1999, Schaller, 2005), by serving as an ischemic preconditioning stimulus and triggering neuroprotective mechanism (Moncaya et al., 2000, Chen et al., 1997). In a retrospective study, Moncayo et al. (2000) reported that TIA of duration no longer than 20 minutes may cover a critical time-period for optimal conditions for subsequent induction of ischemic tolerance in the human brain. It may be concluded therefore that the phenomenon of ischemic tolerance may be also present in patients with ipsilateral TIA before cerebral infarction leading to a better neurological outcome from a subsequent ischemic stroke. These studies do not state that a TIA may prevent a subsequent ischemic event, but if a ischemic event occurs within the same vascular territory and within a limited time window after an appropriate TA, the subsequent ischemic event may be les severe and the neurological recovery better (Weih et al., 1999). In addition, the clinical findings of Moncayo et al. (2000), Weih et al. (1999) and Schaller (2005) underline the assumption that TIA of a duration of less than 10 minutes may less often be followed by ischemic tolerance after a second ischemic event (Moncayo et al., 2000). The favorable clinical recovery after either only one previous ipsilateral TIA or more than three TIAs was comparable to the finding in patients without any previous TIA (Moncoay et al., 2000). From the pathophysiological point of view, Moncayo et al. hypothesized therefore that the duration of ischemia is too short and insufficient to activate the mechanisms involved in ischemic tolerance in patients suffering only one episode, whereas patients with three or more TIAs may demonstrate a cumulative detrimental effects after repeated ischemic events (Moncayo et al., 2000). These clinical findings are comparable and well-known form animal experimental models of focal ischemia, especially when the time-interval between the single episodes is short (Vass et al., 1988; Araki et al., 1990). As shown above, experimentally induced ischemic tolerance is part of a transient phenomenon that needs at least 24 hours to develop after the first brief episode of transient ischemic event (Moncayo et al., 2000). The effect of ischemic tolerance may last approximately 7 days and disappears at the latest after day 14 (Moncayo et al., 2000). Furthermore, patients harboring an interval of 1 week or less between ipsilateral TIA and subsequent cerebral infarction showed a particularly high proportion of favorable neurological recovery, which underlines the hypothesis that ischemic tolerance may be only a transient phenomenon (Moncayo et al., 2000). Leading to the best protective effect against subsequent permanent ischemia, the requested interval between a first TIA and cerebral infarction may therefore be no longer than one week (Moncayo et al., 2000). In addition, it seem that patients with prodromal TIAs display different patterns of diffusion and perfusion deficit in a subsequent stroke (Wegener et al., 2004).

Besides the biochemical explanation in animals, other possibilities such as up-regulated collateral circulation of facilitated thrombolysis, (as observed in the heart (Andreotti et al., 1996)), also must be taken into account in humans (Schaller, 2005). An interesting feature in this context, may be that acetylsalicylic acid (ASA) is neuroprotective independent of its actions on platelets in animal studies (Riepe et al., 1997). It was hypothesized that the protective effect of ASA against hypoxia – at least in part – may be due to a similar increase of endogenous hypoxic tolerance (Riepe et al., 1997). The above-presented clinical data underline this hypothesis.

The traditional concept of TIA adds to this belittlement, although the short-term risk for any adverse event after TIA, either cerebrovascular or cardiovascular, is greater than previously assumed (Rothwell, 2003), and the long-term risk, too, is substantial (Lovett et al., 2003). Because of this and the inability to differentiate TIA from stroke in the hyperacute stage, where thrombolysis is now the state-of-the-art emergency treatment, the term "brain attack" for both, either in combination with cerebral imaging information (Saver, 2004) or not, seems a more adequate approach to improve therapy, mandatory workup, and prediction of prognosis (Daffertshofer et al., 2004). These new findings advocate a new definition or replacement of the term.

2.15.2. Reperfusion

The CBF restoration to ischemic tissues causes additional damage, which is termed reperfusion injury and significantly influences the outcome of patients after ischemic stroke. It is now well accepted that central to ischemic/reperfusion-induced injury is what occurs to mitochondria hours to days following the ischemic insult (Perez-Pinzon et al., 2005). For many years, it has been established that ROS and reactive nitrogen species (RNS) promote lipid, protein, and DNA oxidation that affects normal cell physiology and eventually leads to neuronal demise (Perez-Pinzon et al., 2005). In addition to oxidation of neuronal molecules by ROS and RNS, a novel pathway for molecular modifications has risen from the concept that ROS can activate specific signal transduction pathways that, depending on the insult degree, can lead to either normal plasticity or pathology (Perez-Pinzon et al., 2005). Two examples of these pathways could explain why lethal ischemic insults lead to the translocation of PKC-delta, which plays a role in apoptosis after cerebral ischemia, or why sublethal ischemic insults, such as in ischemic preconditioning, lead to the translocation of epsilonPKC, which plays a pivotal role in neuroprotection (Reshef et al., 2000).

Animal studies indicate that reperfusion injury is reduced by preceding brief periods of ischemia, so-called ischemic preconditioning (Kaeffer et al., 1996; Richard et al., 1994; Thourani et al., 1999). Ischemic preconditioning has direct effects on tissues, making them resistant to ischemic damage but also preventing endothelial dysfunction and inflammatory cell activation associated with reperfusion. These data support the hypothesis that strategies to preserve endothelial function may protect local tissue function and limit reperfusion injury, perhaps by modulating inflammatory cell recruitment (Kharbanda et al., 2001).

Despite convincing data from studies in animals, in humans it remains unclear if endothelial dysfunction occurs during reperfusion injury and whether ischemic preconditioning offers protection against endothelial dysfunction and inflammatory cell activation. The aim of this study was to determine the effects of experimental reperfusion on endothelial and circulating blood cell function in humans in vivo and to examine the neuroprotection afforded by ischemic preconditioning. A better understanding of the mechanisms by which ROS and/or RNS modulate key protein kinases that are involved in signaling pathways that lead to cell death and survival after cerebral ischemia will help devise novel therapeutic strategies (Schaller et al., 2003).

2.15.3. Chronic Mild Reduction of Perfusion Pressure

Leptomeningeal collaterals that may maintain perfusion beyond the site of an arterial occlusion have been appreciated as an important factor both in modifying the size of infarction and in clinical outcome after embolic occlusion of the MCA (Ringelstein et al. 1992; Liebeskind, 2003). Angiogenesis after MCA occlusion has been intensively investigated (del Zoppo et al., 2003; Taguchi et al., 2004). However, little is known about the factors that determine collateral development at the time of embolic occlusion. MCA occlusion has been shown to induce growth and enlargement of surface collaterals in the ischemic border (Wei et al., 2001). Chronic hypoperfusion resulting from extracranial and intracranial occlusive disease promotes leptomeningeal collateral formation, although collaterals require time to develop (Coyle, 1994; Weih et al., 2001; Liebeskind, 2003). The precise role of chronic hypoperfusion in collateral development remains unclear, although it is known that the efficacy of collateral vessels also depends on age, hypertension, and associated comorbidities (Coyle et al., 1991).

Recently, arteriogenesis at the circle of Willis has been demonstrated clearly in a 3-vessel (1 carotid plus both vertebral arteries) occlusion model (Busch et al., 2003). Although reduction of perfusion pressure promotes arteriogenesis at the circle of Willis and in the distal anastomoses that have been described as "pre-existing collateral arterioles" (Buschmann et al., 2000), the diameters of leptomeningeal anastomoses in the 3-vessel occlusion model did not change (Busch et al., 2003). The estimation of vessel diameters may be insufficient for assessing collateral development, particularly in the ischemic condition. Resting cortical perfusion level remained 60% of baseline up to day 28 after common carotid artery (CCA) occlusion (Kitigawa et al., 2005), suggesting us to use a functional evaluation of collateral circulation by measuring the cortical perfusion at the time of MCA occlusion.

The results of Kitigawa et al. (Kitigawa et al., 2005) demonstrate that unilateral CCA occlusion treatment given 14 days before MCA occlusion preserved cortical perfusion and reduced infarct size markedly in the cerebral cortex after MCA occlusion. Negative correlation between changes in perfusion after the first CCA occlusion and at the time of subsequent MCA occlusion in day 14 and day 28 groups suggests that sufficient reduction of perfusion pressure is needed for collateral development (Kitigawa et al., 2005). In general, the development of preexisting collateral arterioles into large conductance vessels may take days to weeks after a critical stenosis of the proximal artery (Buschmann et al., 2000). A direct neuroprotective preconditioning effect after chronic ischemia as shown in the previous study (Ohtsuki et al., 1993) may in part contribute to the effect in day 14 and day 28 groups (Kitigawa et al., 2005). Furthermore, coagulation status such as platelet accumulation and fibrin deposition may change after chronic ischemia as suggested in hypoxia-tolerant states (Stenzel-Poore et al., 2003).

2.16. Remote Preconditioning

During the last few years remote preconditioning, which can be either rapid or delayed has been discovered. In rat brain (Belayev et al., 1996) and rabbit hearts (Takaoka et al., 1999), "remote preconditioning" has been observed, which means that ischemia in the other hemisphere or even in another organ would induce ischemic tolerance. Thus, short episodes of ischemia and reperfusion of the limb (Oxman et al., 1997), colon (Gho et al., 1996), and kidney (Takaoka et al., 1999) may induce ischemic tolerance in other organs as well, and the induction of tolerance may spread via the peripheral nervous system (PNS) or paracrine mechanism to other organs. The underlying mechanisms of remote preconditioning are not clarified, but substances must have been released from the remote ischemic-reperfused tissue that protect the jeopardized brain. Potential neuroprotective substances for an inter-organ transport are (*i*) adenosine, (*ii*) δ1-opiod and (*iii*) neurotransmitters (Przyklenk et al., 2003).

Animal studies have indicated an important role for adenosine receptor activation and subsequent opening of K_{ATP} in this mechanism. Simultaneous activation of the sympathetic nervous system may be involved in so-called "remote" ischemic preconditioning. Up to now, studies on ischemic preconditioning in humans are limited. Important differences between species have been described with respect to the pathophysiology of ischemia and ischemic preconditioning, and this observation underlines the need for further studies on the mechanism of ischemic preconditioning in humans.

2.17. Postconditioning

Brief interruptions (10-60 seconds, depending on the model) of the blood flow applied immediately after the onset of reperfusion following an ischemic event, is observed to provide protection. In the initial study in an anesthetized canine model of coronary artery occlusion-reperfusion, 3 cycles of coronary artery reperfusion alternating with 30 seconds of reocclusion were associated with a significant reduction in both the infarct size and the endothelial dysfunction (Zhao et al., 2003). Similar findings are now also demonstrated in the rat's brain (Zhao et al., 2006). This "postconditioning", so named because the stimulus is applied after the ischemia, is confirmed by others species.

Postconditioning can also be induced via volatile anesthetics (Feng et al., 2005; Weber et al., 2005). Isoflurane, for example, reduced the infract size by 50%, if administered early during reperfusion. Likely, this effect was mediated via the phosphatidylinositol-3 (PI3) kinase (Chiari et al., 2005). Other pharmacological agents administered at the start of reperfusion have been shown to be cardioprotective. These include *(i)* adenosine, *(ii)* NO, *(iii)* cytokine and *(iv)* complement inhibitors. However, whether this approach should be described as "pharmacological postconditioning" or as a "post-reperfusion treatment" has been argued. Since the mechanisms of postconditioning have not been fully elucidated, and the importance of the alternating cycles of ischemia-reperfusion has not been appreciated nor determined to be critical to protecting, direct association to "postconditioning" (whatever "conditioning" means at reperfusion) should be debated.

Experimental studies support the neuroprotective potency of postconditioning to reduce the infarct size, endothelial dysfunction, and neutrophil accumulation in the jeopardized area (Zhao et al., 2006). These experimental results are suggestive that within the first minutes of reperfusion, endogenous processes are initiated that help reduce reperfusion injury after a limited duration of ischemia. The multiplicity of cell types that are affected by postconditioning, i.e. vascular endothelial cells and inflammatory cells, reflects the complexity of reperfusion injury, and suggests a wide network of effects within this complex interactive web of responses.

2.17.1. Mechanisms of Postconditioning

Reperfusion injury is a complex response that involves many of the cells in the integrated structure of the brain. The effects of postconditioning on each of these cell types alone, and then their interaction, must still be described.

It is suggested that limitation of oxygen radicals or of Ca^{2+} overload is involved in the protection. Postconditioning seems to reduce the oxidative stress, in particular by reduction of the superoxide load that is generated, and in mitochondrial peroxide production and the depletion of gluathatione (Serviddio et al., 2005). Other mechanisms to induce postconditioning are guanylyl cyclase activation, opening of the mitochondrial K_{ATP} channels, and inhibiting opening of mitochondrial permeability transition pres (mPTPs) (Feng et al., 2005). Activation of protective pathways (eNOS and NO; ERK1/2; Pl3-kinase – Akt) is also discussed (Vinen-Johansen et al., 2005) as well as adenosine receptors (Kin et al. 2004) and opioid receptors (Kin et al., 2005). Regarding the modulation of these endogenous autacoids, ischemia has been shown to increase the generation of each of these substances. Reperfusion may wash out (adenosine) or reduce the generation (opioids) of these autacoids so that they are no longer available to exert their endogenous cardioprotection. By mechanisms that have not yet been elucidated, postconditioning delays the washout of adenosine, and may thereby increase its exposure to the vascular space in which adenosine may exert potent protection (Todd et al., 1996; Todd et al., 1995). For opioids, postconditioning may promote generation of precursor molecules by unclear mechanisms.

Tsang et al. (Tsang et al., 2004) have proposed that there are "passive" and "active" phases to the mechanisms of postconditioning. The "passive" portion is initiated via stepwise reperfusion that reduces oxygen radicals (presumably the delivery), mitochondrial Ca^{2+} overload, and neutrophils. By the "active" portion, the "reperfusion injury salvage" kinases (RISK) pathway is activated by endogenous stimulators, e.g. adenosine, opioids or other as yet unidentified endogenous substances, and stressors such as ischemia-reperfusion. Here, two interactive pathways might be responsible at least for protection (see Figure 9): (*i*) Activation of PI1 kinase, Akt, and eNOS to inhibit opening of the mPTPs. (*ii*) Activation of MEK1/2 and ERK1/2. In turn, Akt together with ERK1/2 activate p70s6K, which finally initiates protein translation.

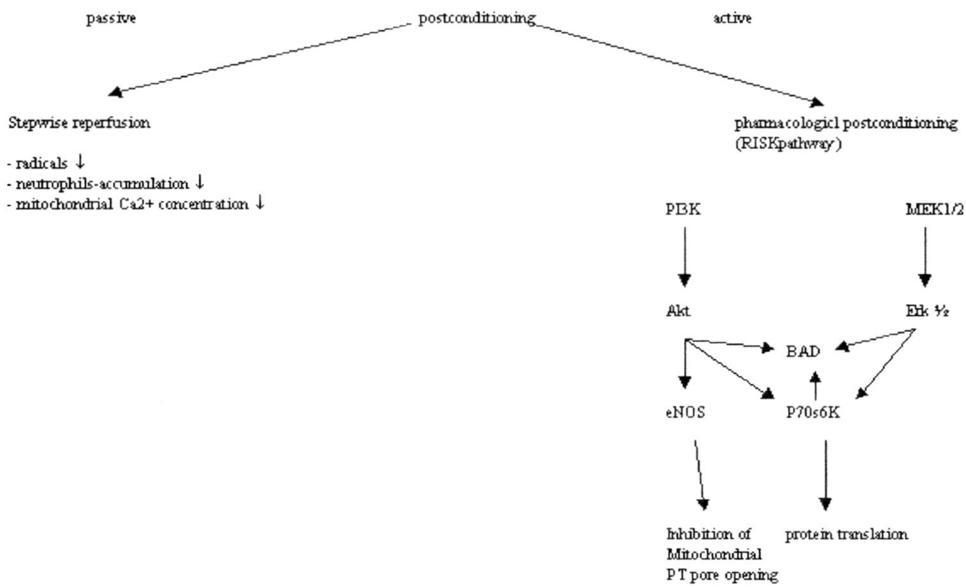

Legend: MEK: mitogen-activated ERK-activating kinase; Erk: extracellular signal-regulated kinase; eNOS: endothelial nitric oxide synthase; PT: permeability transition.

Figure 9. Schematic illustration of postconditioning (modified from Tsang et al., 2004 and Schipke et al., 2006).

In vivo studies to clarify which of the survival kinases are important for postconditioning, suggest that the cardioprotection is likely mediated via the ERK1/2 pathway, rather than via the PI3 kinase/Akt pathway (Darling et al., 2005). An even more recent study comes to the conclusion that in postconditioning both Akt and ERK are activated, but that their activation does not protect from reperfusion injury (Schwarzt et al., 2006). Hence, these early and partially contradictory results need future investigations in models, which isolate the various cell types, and in the integrated organ and organism. In addition, whether there is an active and passive division merits further thought. For example, the "passive" inhibition of neutrophils may be derived from "active" processes of augmenting endogenous signals such as adenosine and opioids, and activation of protein kinase C isoforms that converge on the mPTP, oxidative enzymes and other "effector" targets.

2.17.2. Remote Postconditioning

After having established the term "remote preconditioning", remote postconditioning was experimentally demonstrated as well in the heart: occlusion of the renal artery immediately before the onset of reperfusion of a coronary artery clearly reduced the myocardial infarct size (Kerendi et al., 2005). These investigations provide some results of interest that may be similar in the brain: (*i*) the benefit is likely initiated within the first minutes of the reperfusion of the cerebral artery, (*ii*) the interorgan remote postconditioning is likely mediated via adenosine liberated from the ischemic-reperfused remote organ since neuroprotection is abrogated by an adenosine receptor blocker (8-p-sulfophenyl theophylline). It is not known whether the adenosine receptors were localized in the brain or in a remote organ, and whether neurological mediation of the adenosine stimulus is involved (Kerendi et al., 2005).

The concept of remote preconditioning is not merely a laboratory curiosity; it may have clinical application. One may "stimulate" postconditioning via another organ, such as the leg. This "organ" is much more accessible than the kidney as used in the original study introducing the concept (Kerendi et al., 2005). A tourniquet could be applied to the leg during transport to the emergency room or to the cath-lab to set up a strong postconditioning signal. The tourniquet could then be removed just before completion of the angioplasty procedure and in advance of the onset of reperfusion, being certain to miss the window of neuroprotection afforded in the first minutes of reperfusion (Kin et al., 2004).

Chapter 3

3. Aims of the Study

3.1. Purpose

According to the literature, experimental induced ischemic tolerance correlates with physiological adaptations for ischemic resistance. These adaptations are particularly important in organs that are highly susceptible to energy deprivation such as the heart and brain. Better understanding of the mechanisms inducing both ischemic tolerance or ischemic pre- and postconditioning in mammals may provide novel therapeutic interventions that may aide mammalian brain to resist the ravages of cerebral ischemia. In the light of the increasing interest of cerebral ischemic tolerance not only in experimental, but also clinical neuroscience, it seems to be the time to cumulative present the knowledge with special reference to therapeutic consequences. As postoconditioning seems more clinical applicable, were are the first that planed a postoconditioning study in a best-established animal of cerebral ischemia.

3.2. Main Questions

The following main questions should be answered by the present study:

1. Ischemic tolerance in the brain is yet not well investigated but is different from that in the heart. What may be the biochemical basis of ischemic tolerance in the brain?
2. Has ischemic tolerance that is well documented in experimental models also importance in humans?
3. Can have cerebral postconditioning – that is yet not investigated in the brain - any impact in therapeutic strategies?
4. Is postconditiong effective in every case or only in selected cases?

In order to answer these questions, a prospective animal study was carried out, which included several experimental, anesthesiological and surgical parameters.

Chapter 4

4. Materials and Methods

4.1. Methodology of Literal Research

Medline and Embase databases were searched for trials, case series or case-reports published between 1966 and August 2006 or 1986 and August 2006, respectively. The terms used included *ischemic preconditioning, ischemic tolerance, postconditioning, remote conditioning, cross tolerance, brain, cerebral, anesthetics, erytropoietin, hypothermia, transient ischemic attacks, adenosine receptor, phospholipase, stress proteins, pharamcologicalic preconditioning, thrombin preconditioning, reperfusion, perfusion pressure* and *animal models*. The manuscript had to be published or translated in English, French or German. More recent publications were used in preference to older ones, as the purpose of the review was to give an up-to-date review of the current experimental and clinical knowledge of the role of ischemic tolerance in the brain. Older publications were retried if they were cited in the selected publications and deemed significant for the purposes of this review.

4.2. Animal Preparation

Adult male cats weighting 3.2-4.7 kg were anesthesized with ketamine hydrochloride (25 mg/kg) by intramuscular injection. The left femoral vein and artery were catheterized to measure mean arterial blood pressure (MABP), to obtain samples for determining arterial blood gas levels, hemoglobin, and plasma glucose concentration as well as to administer drugs as necessary. The animals were tracheostomized, immobilized with 0.2 mg/kg pancouronium bromide, and ventilated artificially (FMI, Egelsbach, Germany). Generalized anesthesia was maintained by 0.6-1.2% halothane in a 70% nitrous oxide-30% oxygen gas mixture. An intravenous infusion of 2 ml/kg per h Ringer`s solution containing 5 mg/kg per h gallamine trithiodide for muscle relaxation was maintained throughout the experiments. Physiological variables were kept in the normal range known form awaked cats (Herbert et al., 1971). Deep body temperature was kept at 37° using a heating blanket feedback controlled by a rectal temperature probe.

A large semicoronal skin incision with an additional incision extending posteriorly was made immediately after induction of generalized anesthesia. Subsequently, a myocutaneous flap and a decompressive craniectomy were performed on the left side: a burr hole of 3 mm diameter was drilled fronto-temporally using a dental high-speed drill (Bien Air, Switzerland). For performing a large fronto-temporo-parietal craniectomy (4.5 x 6.0 cm), the temporal squama was rongeured out under microscopic control (Carl Zeiss, Germany) including the following boundaries: anterior, front the midpappilary line; 2 cm posterior to the external auditory meatus; superior 0.5 cm of the lateral edge of the superior sagittal sinus; and inferior, floor of the middle cranial fossa at the origin of the zygomatic arch (to afford adequate decompression of the temporal lobe and middle cranial fossa). Care was taken to avoid lesions of the sigmoid and superior sagittal sinuses (to prevent the possibility of sinus thrombosis). The underlying transparent dura mater was left intact and it was avoided to damage the brain tissue during the procedure.

Subsequent to hemicraniectomy, a cranioplasty was formed to substitute the removed skull. The dura mater was protected with a thin layer of cotton. Methyl methacrylate was prepared in the usual fashion and applied in a semiliquid form onto the underlying brain tissue of the skull defect. After hardening, the cranioplasty and the layer of cotton were removed for definitive remodeling of the cranioplasty. Thereafter, the cranioplasty was reinserted into the skull defect and fixed by suturing without sealing the cranium, and the temporalis muscle and skin flap were adapted and sutured in plane.

A burr hole was made in the left frontoparietal region of the cranioplasty and an intracranial pressure measuring device (Codmann and Shertleff, USA) was placed subdurally on the arachnoidal surface of the marginal gyrus. The burr hole was sealed with methyl methacrylate.

4.3. Positron Emission Tomography Studies

Serial positron emission tomography (PET) scanning was performed with a 24-ring, high resolution camera (Siemens(CTI ECAT EXACT HR) with 207 images plan, an axial field of view of 15 cm, an in-plane spatial resolution of 3.6 mm full width at half maximum and an axial resolution of 4.0 mm full width at half maximum (Wienhard et al., 1985). Starting around 2 hours after hemicraniectomy and cranioplasty, several consecutive PET studies were performed in each cat. For the assessment of cerebral metabolic rate of oxygen (CMRO2) and CBF and cerebral metabolic rate of glucose (CMRGlc), bolus application were used and activity in arterial blood was measured as has been described and discussed before (Baron et al., 1989; Eriksson et al., 1988; Heiss et al., 1994; Heiss et al., 1997; Herscovitch et al., 1983; Minutin et al., 1984; Reivich et al., 1979; Wienhard et al,. 1994).

Transmission scans were acquired with rotating $^{68}Ge/^{68}Ga$ sources and used to correct for photon attenuation. For the assessment of CMRO2, CBF, OEF and CMR_{glc}, bolus applications were used as described elsewhere (Heiss et al., 1994). In brief, 10 mCi $^{15}O_2$ was administered for CMRO2 determination in a single breath by the respirator. CBF was measured after i.v. bolus injection of 20 mCi ^{15}O-labeled water. CMR_{glc} was determined after injection of 5 mCi [^{18}F]fluoro-2-deoxy-D-glucose (FDG) by using regionally estimated rate constants (Wienhard et al. 1994) and a lumped constant of 0.52. Changes of lumped constant in ischemic areas were examined and discussed elsewhere (Gjedde et al. 1985). In areas of low CMRglc, values seem to be underestimated. Experimental background and limitations of these methods for measurement of dynamic alterations of CBF and metabolism have been discussed. Total count rates collected for CBF and CMRO2 studies amounted to 6 and10 million, respectively, in 2-min frames, those for CMR_{glc} studies amounted to 2×10^8 counts in 40-min frames. During $H_2{}^{15}O$ and $^{15}O_2$ scans, activity in arterial blood was measured continuously in an arteriovenous shunt using an automated, calibrated blood-sampling system (Eriksson et al. 1988).

Additionally, three arterial blood samples were taken during $^{15}O_2$ scans for determination of blood gases and for whole-blood and plasma radioactivity measurements and those values were used for parametric image generation. During FDG studies, eight blood samples were taken starting at tracer injection, and plasma radioactivity was used for CMR_{glc} calculations according to the model equation (Reivich et al. 1979).

4.4. Experimental Protocol

To better analyze the outcome in this animal model, we have divided the cats into two subgroups: (*i*) one without prior MCA occlusion ("hemicraniectomy in normal brain") and (*ii*) one with prior MCA occlusion ("decompressive hemicraniectomy after MCA occlusion") before performing the left-sided hemicraniectomy.

4.4.1. Hemicraniectomy in Normal Brain

Routine monitoring of physiological parameters included measurements of heart rate, MABP, rCBF and ICP (for details see Schaller et al., 2004). In addition, end-tidal concentration of CO_2 ($P_{ET}CO_2$; range 3.5-4.5 kPa) and halothane ($P_{ET}HAL$; range 0.8-1.2 kPa) were monitored by use of an infrared gas-analyzer (Datex, Helsinki, Finland). All parameters were continuously recorded using a PC-based data acquisition system (Dasy Lab, National Instruments, USA).

PET images of CBF, CMRO2, and OEF were obtained around 2, 20 and 28 hours after hemicraniectomy, with each multitracer study taking around 20 minutes. CMRGLC (60 minutes) was determined at around 2 and 28 hours after hemicraniectomy. Preceding the last measurements at around 28 hours, the cranioplasty was removed by cutting the holding sutures.

At the end of each experiment, usually 32 hours after hemicraniectomy, animals were perfusion-fixed with formalin (4%), and the brains were removed under maintenance of generalized anesthesia (see Figure 10).

decompressive craniotomy

with intact dura mater and normal brain tissue

↓

cranioplasty

↓

PET at 2 hours postoperative (with cranioplasty):

CBF, CMRO2, OEF, CMRGLC

↓

PET at 20 hours postoperative (with cranioplasty):

CBF, CMRO2, OEF

↓

PET at 28 hours postoperative (without cranioplasty):

CBF, CMRO2, OEF, CMRGLC

Legend: PET: positron emission tomography; CBF: cerebral blood flow; CMRO2: cerebral metabolic rate of oxygen; OEF: oxygen extraction fraction; CMRGLC: cerebral metabolic rate of glucose.

Figure 10. Flow chart of experimental course (adapted from Schaller et al. 2004).

4.4.2. Decompressive Hemicraniectomy after Middle Cerebral Artery Occlusion

The left MCA was exposed transorbitally. A device for remote occlusion (Graf et al., 1986; Ohta et al., 1997) was implanted at the proximal portion of the MCA between the left optic nerve and the MCA bifurcation. The device was completely fixed with gelfoam and rapid-drying glue. Finally, the orbit was sealed with dental cement to avoid CSF leakage and to make again the intracranial space a closed system.

The left MCA was permanently occluded. Decompressive left hemicraniectomy was started 1 hour and completed around 2 hours after MCAO (for details see Graf et al. 2004). Strain gauge microsensors and themorcoulpes implanted on the surface fo the right hemisphre measured ICP and brain temperature throught the experiments.

4.5. Analysis of Positron Emission Tomography Data

Serial PET images were reconstructed using Fourier rebinning and a high-overrelaxation single projection algorithm. Analysis of PET data was based on the parametric images of 16 coronal brain slices. The obtained images permitted the identification of the main anatomic structures of the cat's brain and a distinction of gray and white matter with the best resolution obtained in the CMRGLC images. For quantitative analysis, four regions of interest (ROIs) were defined on 10 consecutive coronal slices enclosing the hemicraniectomy in a stepwise procedure (see figure. 6). The right hemisphere was defined on the first CMRGLC images contralateral to the hemicraniectomy (ROI1). This region was mirrored to the left side forming the region of the left hemisphere (ROI2). In ROI2, a circular region (diameter: 4 mm) was defined on the final CBF image in the center of the CBF defect (ROI4). This circular region was again mirrored to the contralateral side (ROI3). Means of these ROIs were calculated for sequential multiparametric studies.

4.6. Analysis of Histological Data

After paraffin-embedding, serial 7-µm sections (stained with hematoxylin-eosin or Luxol Fast Blue) were obtained in parallel with the PET planes according to a stereotaxic cat brain atlas (Reinoso-Suarez, 1961). The occlusion of the MCAwas verified. Corresponding to the PET slice thickness, serial sections were matched to PET slices and were analyzed at a section-to-section distance of 2 mm for histological verification of infarcts. Areas of ischemic damage in cortex were determined on an image analyzer (Gesotec) under microscopic control and expressed in percentage of cortical areas in the histological sections. Correction for brain swelling was performed. Means of the percentage values of infarction were calculated for individual animals.

4.7. Statistical Analysis

Results are expressed as mean±SD. Statistical analysis was performed using repeated measures. Comparisons between patient groups were analyzed by Student *t* test for quantitative variables, by the Mann-Whitney *U* test for ordinal variables, and by the χ^2 test for categorical variables. ANOVA with Scheffé post-hoc comparison was used to test variation over time and to compare means between left (affected) and right brain hemisphere.

To define a threshold (cutoff value) with optimal diagnostic accuracy for differentiation among groups, we determined the receiver-operating characteristic curve (ROC) and fitted a 45° line on that curve. If sensitivity (ordinate) is plotted versus 1-specificity (abscissa), the best threshold is the point on the ROC that lies on a 45° line closest to the point (0,1) of the ROC plot. Statistical significance was defined at $p<0.05$. Statistical analysis was performed with SPSS for Windows, v. 11 (SPSS).

Chapter 5

5. Results

5.1. General Physiological Parameters

Arterial blood gas levels, pH and hemoglobin concentration in the cats remained within normal physiological limits throughout the experiments. Both mean systemic arterial pressure and intracranial pressure were not significantly altered by the surgical procedure (hemicraniectomy followed by cranioplasty), by the removal of the cranioplasty, nor in the later course of the experiments.

5.2. Positron Emission Tomography Measurements

5.2.1. Hemicraniectomy in Normal Brain

PET scans obtained around 2 hours after hemicraniectomy are illustrated on coronal planes in figure 6 (for details see Schaller et al., 2003). The surgical procedure decreased CBF ($p<0.01$) and increased OEF ($p<0.05$) significantly in regions of the left hemisphere underneath the hemicraniectomy. In contrast, CMRO2 and CMRGLC were not affected.

Evaluation of means in both hemispheres and in the two circular regions revealed that CBF decreased in brain tissue regions below the hemicraniectomy (see Figure 11). Comparison of the tow sides showed that the decrease of CBF amounted to 20-30% of the contralateral hemisphere in the center planes 4-7 of the defect (see evaluation of circular regions in Figure 12). The larger percent decrease of CBF in the circular regions reflects the more focused regional analysis.

Further data analysis of all PET parameters over time was focused on these four center planes to particularly provide a sensitive test for alterations of metabolic parameters, i.e., CMRO2 and CMRGLC (see Figure 13). Initial decreased of CBF in these four center planes remained almost unchanged over the entire experimental period of around 1 day. A slight tendency of further deterioration of blood flow may be recognized at the second time point on day 2 (20 hours), but subsequent removal of the cranioplasty did not have any additional effect. Comparing the means of regions of interest in the two hemispheres, neither metabolic parameters showed significant changes. Alterations of metabolic parameters over time were minimal, if existent, and these alterations were also not significant.

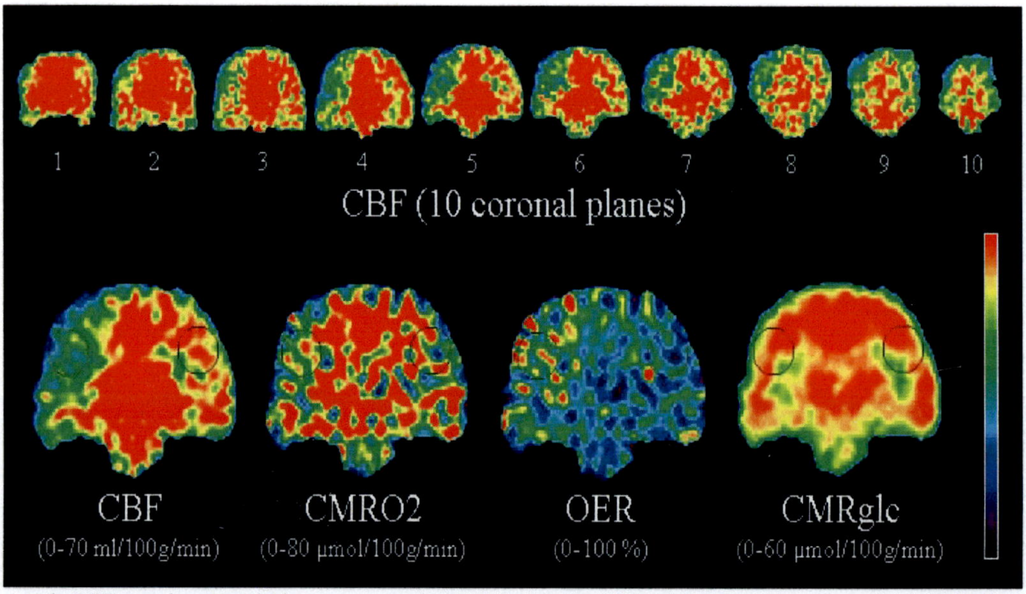

Legend: PET: positron emission tomography; CBF: cerebral blood flow; CMRO2: cerebral metabolic rate of oxygen; OEF: oxygen extraction fraction; CMRGLC: cerebral metabolic rate of glucose.

Figure 11. PET images taken around 2 hours after hemicraniectomy. Upper row: 10 consecutive coronal planes of CBF. Lower row. Comparisons of CBF, CMRO2, OEF, and CMRGLC of plane 5.

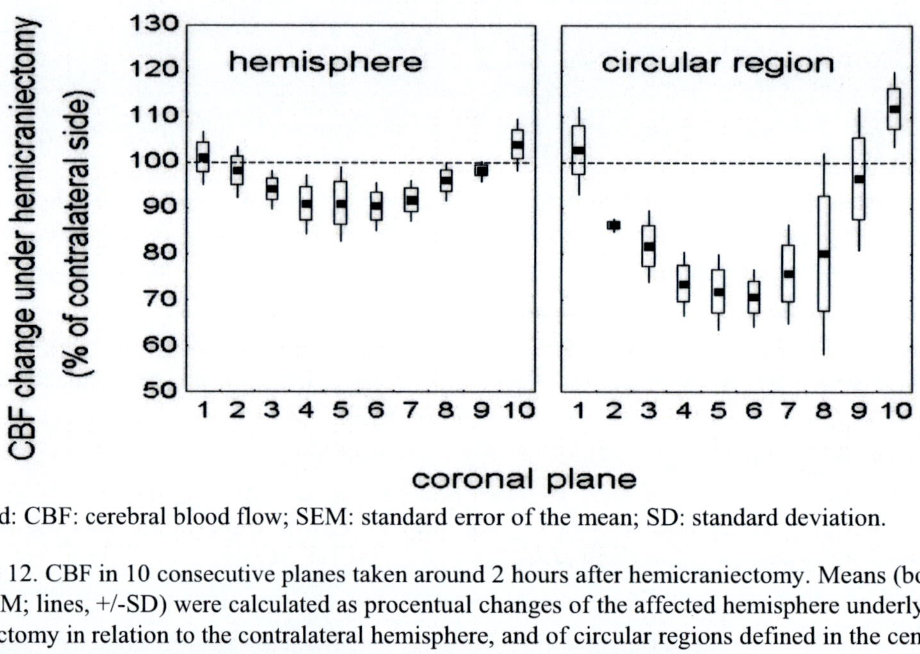

Legend: CBF: cerebral blood flow; SEM: standard error of the mean; SD: standard deviation.

Figure 12. CBF in 10 consecutive planes taken around 2 hours after hemicraniectomy. Means (boxes, +/- SEM; lines, +/-SD) were calculated as procentual changes of the affected hemisphere underlying the craniectomy in relation to the contralateral hemisphere, and of circular regions defined in the center of the effect in relation to mirror circular regions in the contralateral hemisphere.

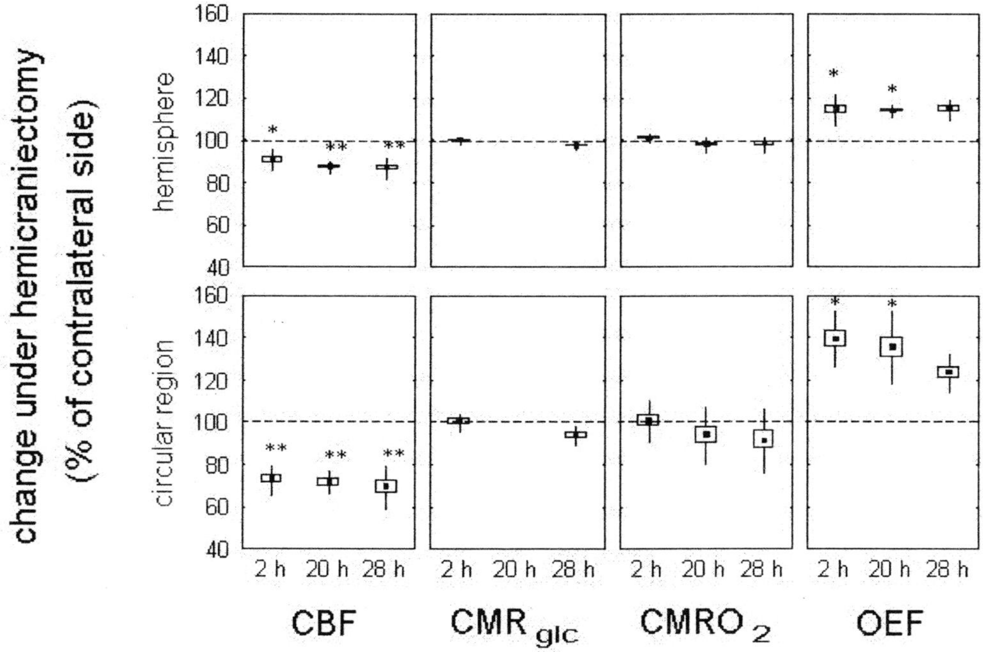

Legend: SEM: standard error of the mean; SD: standard deviation; PET: positron emission tomography; CBF: cerebral blood flow; CMRO2: cerebral metabolic rate of oxygen; OEF: oxygen extraction fraction; CMRGLC: cerebral metabolic rate of glucose.

Figure 13. CBF, CMRGLC, CMRO2 and OEF in four center planes (planes 4-7, see figure 7): 2, 20 and 28 hours after hemicraniectomy. Means (boxes, +/- SEM; lines, +/- SD; * $p<0.05$, ** $p>0.01$) were calculated as percentual changes of the affected hemisphere underlying the craniectomy in relation to the contralateral hemisphere, and of circular regions defined in the center of the effect in relation to mirror circular regions in the contralateral hemisphere.

The means of OEF, in contrast, were significantly changed by the surgical procedure. Additional changes of OEF over time and due to removal of the cranioplasty were not significant.

To attain a higher sensitivity regarding effects of craniectomy on metabolic parameters, we plotted means of CMRO2 and CMRGLC of the left circular regions in the four center planes (as percent of regions in the right hemisphere) against corresponding means of CBF (see Figure 14). Surprisingly, these correlations were positive documenting that at least in regions with most severe CBF reductions, metabolism was reduced. This effect was clearer for oxygen ($R=0.75$; $p<0.05$) that for glucose metabolism ($r=0.64$; $p<0.05$).

The fact that means of CMRO2 and CMRGLC ranged between around 70-120% and 85-110%, respectively, obscured this relationship, because resulting means did not significantly deviate from values obtained in the hemisphere contralateral to the craniectomy. The correlation of CBF with OEF was negative ($r=0.24$; p n.s.) as expected from the main regional analysis, but less pronounced. This may be a result of the larger scatter that is generally obtained in PET images of OEF.

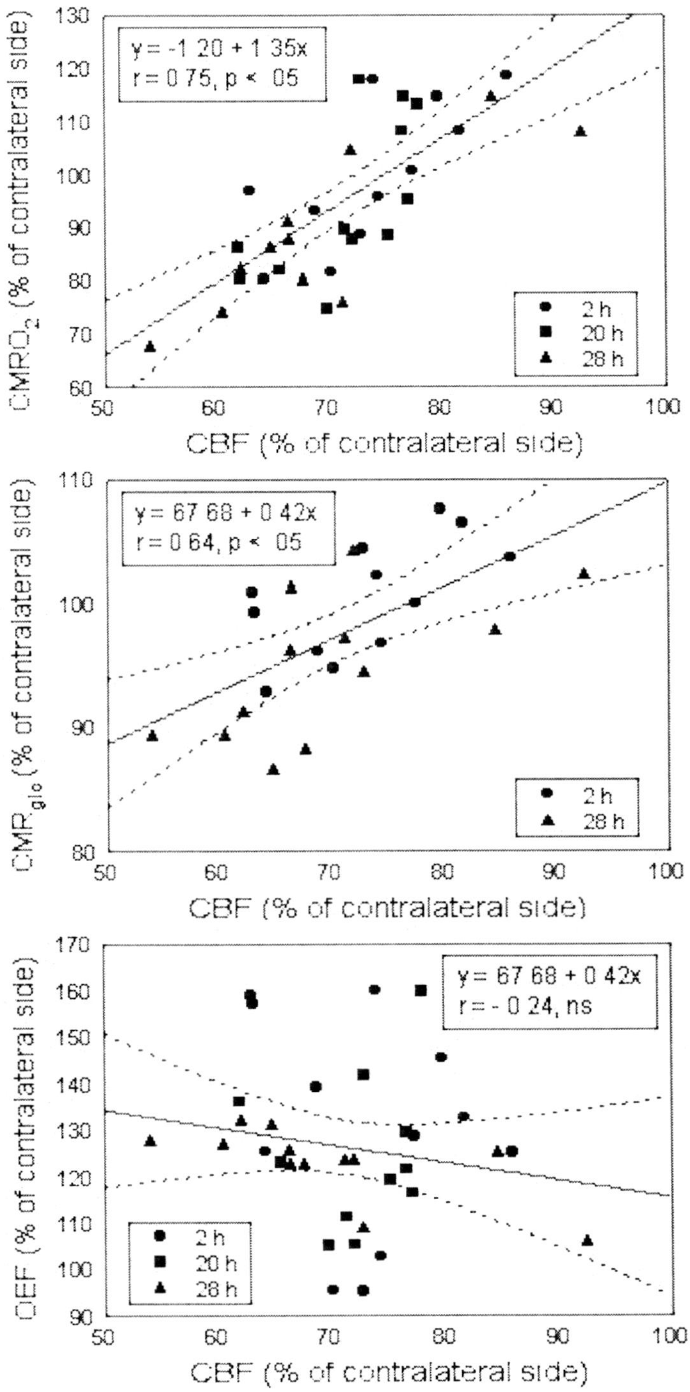

Figure 14. Diagram of CBF related to CMRO2 (upper), CMRGLC (middle), and OEF (lower), and corresponding linear regression lines with 5% confidence interval.

5.2.2. Decompressive Hemicraniectomy after Middle Cerebral Artery Occlusion

MCAO reduced PET-CBF in all animals. The effects of hemicraniecotmy, in contrast, varied among the animals. Thirty per cent of animals showed pronounced recovery of CBF in parts of the ischemic territory that lasted until next day. In the other cats, this event was less pronounced. Pixel by pixel analysis showed that (*i*) the ischemic territory after MCAO (CBF < 20 ml/100g/min) decreased immediately after hemicraniectomy by 27 +/- 10% compared to that that during and that (*ii*) mean CBF values in ischemic territories decreased to 38+/- 22% of contralateral after MCAO, increased to 46 +/- 18% immediately following hemicraniectomy, but decreased again to 28 +/- 13% on next day.

Chapter 6

6. Discussion

The present study was able to demonstrate for the first time by sequential PET images that early decompressive hemicraniectomy after MCAO improved CBF transiently and showed occurrence of ischemic tolerance. This overall effect was significant, but variation among individual animals is pronounced. This study gives different interesting features on ischemic tolerance, (*i*) demonstrating – for the first time – that hemicraniectomy after stroke may set postconditioning stimuli that improve early outcome and (*ii*) giving evidence that hemicraniectomy may substantially improve the time window for further therapeutic options. But our study demonstrates that hemicraniectomy represents an invasive treatment option and indicates that this procedure may provide long-lasting benefit to the ischemia-threatened tissue only in individual cases.

6.1. Time Window

Time between ischemic injury and start of therapy is often discrepant between preclinical and clinical studies. Therapeutic manipulations generally work best when administered before and immediately after the insult (Danton et al., 2004). Experiments with animal models often begin with such a pretreatment protocol. If the therapy works, it is tested at different intervals from injury onset. Most effective therapies work best within 15–30 minutes; rarely are they effective more than 3 hours after injury (Grotta et al., 1999). Although there is little reason to assume the therapeutic window in small animals relates to the window in humans, less than 3 hours seems to fit both paradigms. Unfortunately, it is difficult to get patients to the hospital, evaluated, and enrolled in a clinical trial within 3 hours of symptom onset (Danton et al., 2004). More than 17,324 patients were screened to enroll the 624 subjects in the National Institute of Neurological Disorders and Stroke (NINDS) recombinant tissue-type plasminogen activator (t-PA) trial, and most were excluded because of the time window (Gladstone et al., 2002; The National Institute of Neurological Disorders and Stroke rt-PA Stroke Study Group, 1995). In the European Cooperative Acute Stroke Study II, which looked at recombinant t-PA therapy with a treatment window between 0 and 6 hours, more than 80% of patients were treated between 3 and 6 hours and no effect was detected (Hacke et al., 1995). Had the

NINDS trial chosen a longer window, a difference might not have been detected and recombinant t-PA might not have made it to clinical use. To avoid erroneously discarding a beneficial therapy, future trials should either strictly enforce enrollment or stratify patients into groups based on time-to-treat. Conducting randomized, double-blind, placebo-controlled studies that stratify patients based on time-to-treat will require larger numbers of subjects and take longer to complete; however, these studies may give investigators the best chance of detecting efficacious therapies.

Preclinical studies often begin with a pretreatment design to improve chances of detecting an effect. Clinical correlates to pretreatment studies include administering neuroprotective agents to long-term high-risk patients or during procedures that carry risk of stroke such as carotid endarterectomy or those involving the aortic arch. Most procedures have relatively small risks of complications, so these studies would likely take a long time to acquire sufficient numbers of subjects but may help establish the neuroprotective potential of new therapeutics. We present here an animal model that imitates the clinical requirements as good as possible (Schaller et al., 2004) and can explain to underlying mechanism of hemicraniectomy and can give substantial experimental evidence that patient selection may be of outmost importance to achieve the suspected therapeutic goal.

6.2. Postconditioning vs. Preconditioning

Postconditioning provides neuroprotective effects similar to ischemic preconditioning (Zhan et al., 2003). Comparison of postconditioning and preconditioning exhibits relatively many similarities (see table 8). Studies on different species demonstrated that both phenomena reduced the infarct area to similar degrees and protected vascular endothelial function (Vinten-Johnansen et al., 2005). Our study demonstrates for the first time that postconditioning of the brain may have effects in stroke therapy, even so the underlying mechanisms are not fully understood.

Already in the "preconditioning area", the question was asked whether or not multiple triggers could enhance neuroprotection (Schaller et al., 2003). However, an additive effect could exist for preconditioning plus postconditioning. Yet, in a study on anesthetized dogs, postconditioning did not amplify protection beyond the preceding preconditioning (Halkos et al, 2004). This finding suggests that the injury due to reperfusion can be reduced. It is still not clear whether the two neuroprotective strategies are additive under certain circumstances, such as prolonged ischemia in which the protection of one or the other maneuver drops out (Gumina et al., 1999). If the two maneuvers do indeed share identical mechanisms, then they may not be additive unless tow "bouts" are better than one. Certainly, it is not known whether multiple episodes of postconditioning spread out over the early and later phases of reperfusion are neuroprotective, although a number of cycles within each episode does not seem important. On the other hand, if there are differences in the molecular mechanisms (i.e. ERK1/2 vs. PI3-kinase) or the timing of effect (ischemia vs. reperfusion) then the two maneuvers may be additive under the correct circumstances.

Table 8. Comparison between preconditioning and postconditioning (adapted from Vinten-Johanson et al., 2005 and Schipke et al., 2006)

		Prec-con	Post-con
(i) Physiologigical Effects			
reduces	infarct size	+	+
	apoptosis	+/-	+ (?)
	tissue edema	+	+
	vascular injury	+	+
	endothelial dysfunction	+	+
	perfusion injury	+	+
delays	adenosine washout	-	+
(ii) Cellular and Subcellular Effects			
inhibits	neutrophil accumulation	+	+
	neutrophil-attachment on endothelial cells	+	+
	endothelial cell activation	+	+
	O_2-generation by endothelial cells	+	+
	O_2-generation by myocytes	+	+
	generation of cytokines	+	?
activates	K_{ATP} channel	+	+
closes	mitochondria	+	+
	permeability transition pores	+	+
mediated via	adenosine	+	+
	opiods	+	+
(iii) Molecular Effects			
pathways	PI3 kinase/pAkt	+	+/-
	GSK3β	+	?
	ERK ½-MEK	-	+
	P70S6K	+	+
	eNOS	+	+

Legend: pre-con: preconditioning; post-con: postconditioning; K_{ATP} channel: ATP-sensitive K^+channels; GSK: Glycogen synthase kinase; ERK: extracellular signal-regulated kinase; eNOS: endothelial nitric oxide synthase.

6.3. Controversies in the Experimental and Clinical Application of Preconditioning

The mechanisms of preconditioning have been best studied in the heart and brain. These cellular mechanisms and protective strategies are still developing in other organs, including the lung. There are still many controversies on the effects of preconditioning for the following reasons (Schulz et al., 2001) making more related researches necessary. (*i*) Preconditioning phenomena has differences among species. For example, the functional role for PKC isoenzymes differs among species, with PKCε being most important in rabbits, PKCδ in rats and PKCα in dogs. It appears that results from large mammals are closer to those from humans. (*ii*) Different experimental models (in vitro versus in vivo, anesthetized versus conscious animals) will affect the results. (*iii*) The age of the animals or human beings will also affect the results. (*iv*) Modes of preconditioning, such as the cycles and duration of the preconditioning stimuli, low flow vs. no flow and regional vs. global ischemia will also affect the results. The site of blockade (redundant or non-redundant signaling pathway) will also yield different results. (*v*) The results of pharmacological agents are valuable tools for discovering the mechanisms of preconditioning. However, the results will be influenced by the effectiveness and specificity of the drugs for a given target at a given concentration. (*vi*) The intraspecies differences, the rate of transfection, the redundancy of the signaling pathway should be considered in experiments on transgenic or transfective approaches.

6.4. Therapeutic Implications of Ischemic Tolerance

6.4.1. Preconditioning

A fundamental question in translating results of animal experiments to clinical use is whether or not the pathophysiologic processes in animal models correlate with those in human disease. Differences may arise from (*i*) differences in anatomy and physiology, (*ii*) differences in pathophysiologic response to injury, or (*iii*) differences between injury mechanisms in animal models and those in human disease. The first two problems have been addressed by using multiple species in each model. As a therapy advances toward clinical trials, larger animals, including primates, may be used to better predict response in humans. The third problem can be addressed by testing therapeutics in multiple models. Therapies that work in many models are more likely to target fundamental pathomechanisms and apply to human disease. Unfortunately, investigators often gain expertise in only a few similar models with questionable applicability to human disease. Furthermore, having multiple, independent laboratories replicate studies provides a stronger rationale for moving a therapy to the clinic as the probability of having multiple false-positive studies are reduced.

Neuroprotective strategies can be divided into those that limit the ischemic cascade or those that reduce reperfusion injury (see Figure 15). Neurons die under ischemic conditions when delivery of oxygen and an energy source (i.e., glucose) are not sufficient to meet their metabolic demands. Therefore, ischemic neurons must either receive increased blood flow or their metabolic demands need to decrease. The most important step in limiting ischemia is the quick restoration of CBF that occurs either naturally or with the aid of thrombolytic substances. Before complete restoration of CBF, therapies such as hypothermia may decrease metabolic demand (Erecinska et al., 2003) and extend neuron survival (Wassmann et al., 1998). Once depleted of energy, membrane-bound ion pumps fail, leading to membrane depolarization, Na^+ and Ca^{2+} entry, and neurotransmitter release (Taylor et al., 1995). Dendritic glutamate release activates downstream neurons, leading to calcium entry, cellular damage, apoptosis, and further release of toxic molecules.

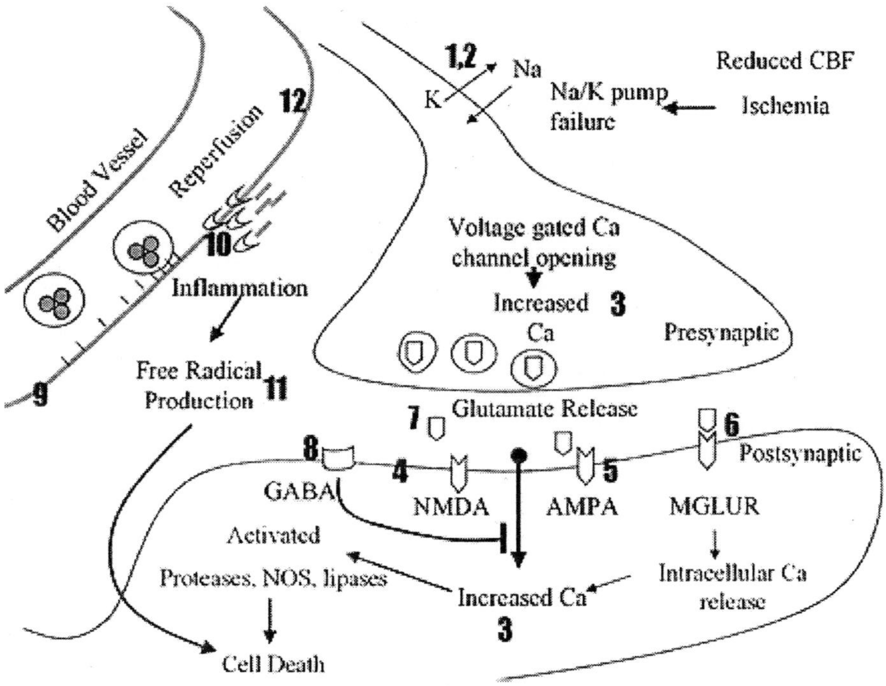

Legend: When the presynaptic neuron becomes ischemic, it depolarizes, opening sodium (Na^+) and potassium (K^+) channels (1, 2). This leads to opening of calcium (Ca^{2+}) channels and influx of calcium (3). The presynaptic cell releases glutamate that activates N-methyl-D-aspartic acid (NMDA), α-amino-5-hydroxy-3-methyl-4-isoxazole propionic acid (AMPA), and metabotropic glutamate receptors (MGLURs) (4–6), which permits calcium entry in the postsynaptic cell. N-acetylated alpha-linked acidic dipeptidase (NAALADase) inhibitors limit the amount of glutamate available for release (7). Gamma-aminobutyric acid (GABA) agonists inhibit depolarization and prevent calcium entry (8). During reperfusion, upregulated adhesion molecules attract inflammatory cells that contribute to vessel occlusion and cytotoxin production (9). Matrix metalloproteinase (MMPs) degrade the basement membrane around vessels, enhancing inflammation and edema (10). Inflammatory cells, ischemic neurons, and glia produce free radicals that contribute to cell damage and death (11). 3-hydroxy-3-methylglutaryl-CoA (HMG-CoA) reductase inhibitors (statins) stabilize the endothelium through upregulation of endothelial nitric oxide synthase (NOS, 12).

Figure 15. The ischemic cascade (with permission of G. Danton, USA).

Agents that modulate ion channels and glutamate receptors target this pathway (Ovbiagele et al., 2003; Jain et al., 2000). Reperfusion injury was observed by comparing infarct volumes in animal models of transient and permanent ischemia (Nakayama et al., 1988; Watson et al., 1987). Reperfusion, while critical to limit ischemia, contributes to cell death by enhancing production of free radicals, inflammation, and BBB breakdown; each has been targeted by therapies (Ovbiagele et al., 2003; Jain, 2000; Clark et al., 1999; Carden et al., 2000).

Clinically, the most effective breakthrough in the treatment of cerebral ischemia has been the successful establishment of systemic thrombolysis (Heiss et al., 1997). With the increasing knowledge about the dynamics of pathophysiological and molecular mechanisms leading to ischemia-related cell damage and about the presumed molecular targets of treatments counteracting these mechanisms, combinatorial treatment strategies based on thrombolysis and endogenous neuroprotection have to be developed. Ischemic tolerance seems to be a very strong candidate in serving a better understanding of the molecular mechanisms involved in neuroprotection as well as in improving therapeutic strategies for patients with stroke or other ischemia-related diseases.

The combination of reperfusion by either thrombolytic or fibrinolytic agents with endogenous neuroprotectants may offer significant advantages to the singular use of each strategy (Aranowski et al., 1996). Thus, reperfusion may be associated with excessive production of reactive oxygen species in the previously ischemic areas and this may contribute to further tissue damage (Ashwal et al., 1998; Endres et al., 1998). Adjuvant (endogenous) neuroprotective agents may help to reduce such damage and therefore, increase the therapeutic gain of reperfusion (Bowes et al., 1995). Furthermore, reperfusion may enhance the therapeutic effect of neuroprotective agents due to better delivery into the ischemic region.

The value of hypothermic preconditioning in the clinical setting clearly remains to be established. However, the findings presented in this chapter indicate that the clinical evaluation of preconditioning may be warranted. In particular, hypothermia exhibits several desirable features of a candidate mechanism for inducing tolerance: (*i*) noninvasive treatment, (*ii*) although not without side effects, hypothermia-induced tolerance is expressed, and declines, over a manageable time course, and (*iii*) hypothermia is already in use clinically as an intraischemic and postischemic therapy. Implementations of this strategy could yield substantial benefit in the context of predictable ischemia, such as occurs in a wide variety of common surgical procedures.

6.4.2. Anesthetics

Accumulating evidence indicates that anesthetics might be beneficial to injured brain. Barbiturates, propofol, benzodiazepines, ethmoidate, and most inhalational anesthetics (halothane, isoflurane, sevoflurane, desflurane, xenon) have proven to cause major reduction in cerebral metabolic rate and induced neuroprotection in animals.

In a model of incomplete hemispheric ischemia, Baughman et al. (Baughman et al., 1988) demonstrated neuroprotection in rats anesthetized with isoflurane or halothane. Warner et al (Warner et al., 1993) demonstrated the neuroprotective effect of halothane or sevoflurane during focal cerebral ischemia in rats. After cardiac arrest in dogs, isoflurane reduces damage of the hippocampal neurons (Blanck et al., 2000). Miura et al. (Miura et al., 1998) provided evidence that protection against neuronal injury by isoflurane during near-complete ischemia is superior to protective effects of fentanyl or ketamine anesthesia. In a recent publication, Bhardwaj et al. (Bhardwaj et al., 2001) presented data on neuroprotection with halothane anesthesia after focal cerebral ischemia induced immediately after the termination of anesthesia.

All these studies used volatile anesthetics shortly before and during the ischemic period. However, it is also known that volatile anesthetics can induce the expression of several genes belonging to the class of immediate-early genes (IEGs), and this effect is not restricted to nervous tissue only (Marota et al., 1992; Hamaya et al., 2000). IEGs are transcription factors induced as a stress response and are implicated in ischemic tolerance induction in the brain (Yoneda et al., 1997; Kapinya et al., 2000). Thus, induction of IEGs is expected to lead to long-lasting changes in the expression of various gene products.

This leads to the hypothesis that the well-described neuroprotection during general anesthesia might not be restricted to the duration of anesthesia but may be sustained long after anesthesia has been terminated.

Numerous explanations for the acute neuroprotective effects of volatile anesthetics have been discussed in the literature. Blockade of ischemia-induced glutamate release (Patel et al., 1995), induction of γ-aminobutyric acid type A receptor–associated K^+ influx (Quinlan et al., 1995; Shuaib et al., 1996), and inhibition of *N*-methyl-D-aspartate gated ion channels (Yang et al., 1991) might all be involved in neuroprotection by anesthetics. However, all the available studies focused on the direct effects of anesthesia and did not investigate the effects many hours after anesthesia. Because volatile anesthetics, and especially isoflurane, are poorly metabolized and rapidly washed out of the organism (Carpenter et al., 1986), it is very likely that the delayed effects (>12 hours after administration) reported in the present study do not involve the presence of the agent. This conclusion is further strengthened by the fact that isoflurane also induces delayed neuroprotection in neuronal cultures. In cell culture, the washout of compounds via the gas space and multiple medium changes is greatly facilitated by the very large ratio of extracellular to intracellular space.

It is interesting to note that activator proteins (AP) differ from other previously reported models of ischemic preconditioning. In other models of induced tolerance to ischemia, there is a time window in which there is no protection against ischemia: 12 to 14 hours between the early phase of induced tolerance (which occurs within minutes and subsides within hours) and the delayed phase, which is manifested after 24 hours (and is maintained for days). Kainya et al. believe that the continuum of protection of AP is mediated by various mechanisms that overlap in time to produce the sustained level of protection (Kainya et al., 2002). This is also suggested by the inducible nitric oxide synthase (iNOS) expression data in the present study, inasmuch as iNOS expression increases only 6 hours after AP, whereas protection was already present immediately after AP. Therefore, the early phase of protection cannot be attributed to iNOS but is more likely due to the acute effect of anesthesia, as discussed below.

Surprisingly little attention has been paid so far to the effects of volatile anesthetics on gene expression. The few studies available focused on the members of the IEG family of transcription factors, especially on c-*fos*. Induction of c-*fos* and *jun-B* in the rat brain after pentobarbital and halothane anesthesia has been demonstrated by Marota et al. (Marota et al., 1992). In an immunohistochemical study, Takayama et al (Takayama et al., 1994) demonstrated the induction of c-*fos* expression as its protein product by various anesthetic agents. The observed changes in gene expression imply that some phenotypical alterations may remain even after cessation of the anesthetic effect. Identification of target genes that are controlled by IEGs might reveal the molecular mechanisms underlying the late effect of volatile anesthetic treatment. Positive findings in the literature linking iNOS or NO to prolonged protection against ischemia tempted us to select iNOS as a potential candidate for transmitting AP (Takano et al., 1998; Guo et al., 1999; Leesar et al., 2001; Gonzalez-Zulueta et al., 2000). We found a significant induction of iNOS protein expression in the cerebral cortex, and inhibition of iNOS abolished the effect of AP. The possibility that nitric oxide (NO) is critically involved in protective signaling in the brain is supported by several other reports. NO was found to be involved in the function of the p21^{ras}/extracellular signal–regulated kinase cascade, which, in turn, was found to be necessary for ischemic tolerance induction in neuronal cell culture (Gonzalez-Zulueta et al., 2000). NO suppresses nuclear factor-κB–mediated gene expression (Togashi et al., 1997). Furthermore, nitroxyl anion (NO^-) has been shown to interact with the NR2A subunit of the *N*-methyl-D-aspartate receptor, with a subsequent reduction of Ca^{2+} influx (Kim et al., 1999). NO^- can be formed from NO by interfering with redox metal–containing proteins in physiological systems. Thus, involvement of iNOS or NO in AP is likely, but further investigation is needed to elucidate the complete pathway.

6.4.3. Postconditioning

Parallel with certain euphoria, criticism about the relatively young phenomenon "postconditioning" exists. E.g. postconditioning could simply be a from of stepwise/controlled reperfusion (Heusch et al., 2004), which is already is under clinical circumstances in the heart. On the other hand, this form of reperfusion could present a valuable strategy in cerebral bypass surgery to reduce cerebral ischemic injury. However, it is not clear at this early point how postconditioning differs from other forms of modified reperfusion such as "gradual reperfusion", if at all. There are some interesting differences between the tow modes of reperfusion. This in itself is a potential field of investigation.

Before any routine use in the clinic, one should keep in mind that hearts might be preconditioned already via repeat TIA episodes or by anesthetics. Thus, additional neuroprotection may not be expected. If required, postconditioning could be initiated via appropriate anesthetics (Chiari et al., 2005). After all, postconditioning may be superior to preconditioning as protective interventions after ischemic stroke can easily performed (Zhang et al., 2006).

6.5. Prospect to the Future

6.5.1. Preconditioning

If a multifaceted and coordinated genetic program involving the expression of multiple genes in neurons, glia and endothelial cells guides ischemic tolerance, it seems unlikely that such a complex endogenous genetic response could be mimicked by a single neuroprotective drug (Fisher et al., 2003). One way to identify transcription factors specific for ischemia and ischemic tolerance is to find common DNA regulatory element(s) in the promoter regions of the genes that are up-regulated in distinct cell types by ischemic tolerance (DeGracia et al., 2002). Identification of these sequences as well as transcriptions factors that bind to them could represent the class of future molecular targets and novel drugs. Small molecules capable of activating transcription factors induced by ischemia could augment an endogenous protective response such as ischemic tolerance. If a class of transcriptional activators could be identified in humans, this would open a window into guided endogenous neuroprotection and possibly also towards further developments to utilize these mechanisms in the treatment of acute stroke and other central nervous system disorders. For example, since over-expression of Hsp 70 results in cell that are more resistant to various stresses, Hsp70 gene transfer has been successfully employed to abrogate ischemic damage (Yenari et al., 1998).

A clear understanding of the mechanism involved in either form of ischemic protection (early or late) is essential to allow a reasoned approach to novel drug design (see table 9). With an appropriate time interval, application of a mild dosage of selective inhibitors of mitochondrial complex I or mitochondrial complex II increases primary hypoxic tolerance – ischemic preconditioning respectively. Preconditioning by pharmacological agents has been studied most extensively with 3-nitropropianate, an inhibitor of succinic dehyodrogenase (Riepe et al., 1997; Riepe et al., 1996).

Table 9. Major proposed pharmacological substances for induction of ischemic preconditioning

(i) Chaperon Inducer

-hydroxylamine derivate (Vigh et al., 1997)

-gernylgeraylacetone (Hirakawa et al., 1996)

(ii) Hematological Factors

-erythopoetin (Dawson, 2002)

(iii) Sucinic Dehydrogenase Inhibitor

-3-nitropropionic acid (Riepe et al., 1996)

(iv) Antibiotics

-erythomycin (Huber et al., 1999)

-kanamycin (Huber et al., 1999)

(v) Non-metabolitable Analog of Glucose

-2-deoxyglucose (Gonzalez-Zulueta et al., 2000)

(vi) Prostaglandin Synthethase Antagonist

-acetylsalicylic acid (Riepe et al., 1997)

(vii) NMDA Receptor Anatagonist

-MK-801 (Gonzalez-Zuleta et al., 2000)

(viii) NO synthethase Antagonist

-L-nitroarginine methyl ester (Gonzalez-Zuleta et al., 2000; Yu et al., 1999)

Legend: NMDA: N.methyl-D-aspartate; NO: nitric oxide.

Recently, it was suggested that chemic-pharmacological induction of preconditioning is unknowingly already in use (Riepe et al., 1997): ASA, which is the most widely used drug for secondary stroke prevention, is known to inhibit mitochondrial energy metabolism (Whitehouse et al., 1962). Although the time course of action and the gender specific effects of the effectiveness of acetylsalicylate cannot be explained in terms of inhibition of platelet aggregation, it possibly can be explained within the paradigm of preconditioning (Riepe et al., 1997).

Even with the development of pharmacological agents that can mimic or evoke ischemic preconditioning, the timing of administration will be critical. Prompt reperfusion will always remain the most effective method of limiting ischemic injury and is, therefore, the most important determinant of prognosis. However, there are certain clinical situations in which the timing of treatment before the onset of ischemia can be controlled to some extent. Prophylactic neuroprotection would include (*i*) short-term neuroprotection before and after high-stroke risk procedures, (*ii*) long-term neuroprotection for primary and secondary intervention in populations at high risk for stroke, and (*iii*) concomitant neuroprotection with agents that have multiple treatment effects (Schaller et al., 2003).

In future, this may include a specific chemo-pharmacological induction of ischemic tolerance in small subgroups of patients before surgical interventions with a high risk of hypoxia or ischemia, as endarterctomy of cerebral carotid artery or cerebral aneurysm surgery. Several populations at high long-term risk for initial ischemic stroke have been identified and include those with combinations of vascular risk factors, TIA, atrial fibrillation, and asymptomatic carotid stenosis (Fisher et al., 1995). Such people, as well as those at risk for stroke recurrence after minor strokes, are readily identifiable and perhaps appropriate for long-term prophylactic neuroprotection.

6.5.2. Postconditioning

Previous studies described considerable species depending differences. On the other hand, preconditioning and ponstconditioning induced comparable protection but to different genomic responses. Thus, for longer periods, beneficial effects could be different (Lucchinetti et al., 2005). Since the underlying mechanism of postconditioning remain unclear, much rooms is left for future studies.

Chapter 7

7. Conclusion

A brief episode of ischemia renders the brain more resistant against subsequent, longer ischemic episodes. This so called ischemic tolerance has been shown in numerous experimental models of cerebral ischemia. Although the exact mechanism of ischemic tolerance in the brain remains uncertain, its discovery years ago provides the focus for a further understanding of the mechanisms of endogenous neuroprotection and the potential of novel therapeutic strategies for neuroprotection. The current experimental research focused on the factors which enable the brain to enter a hypometabolic state, including decreases in ion flux ("channel arrest"), increases in inhibitory neuromodulators like adenosine and GABA, and the maintenance of low extracellular levels of excitatory compounds such as dopamine and glutamate. Our attention has recently turned to molecular mechanisms of cerebral ischemic tolerance, including the up-regulation of such neuroprotective factors as heat shock proteins, the reversible down-regulation of voltage gated potassium channels, and the modulation of MAP kinase pathways. There was hypothesized three phases of cerebral ischemia tolerance, including (*i*) the initial metabolic down-regulation over the first several hours, (*ii*) the long-term maintenance of neuronal function over days to weeks of anoxia, and finally (*iii*) recovery upon reoxygenation, with necessary defenses against reactive oxygen stress. The questing of timing of the "conditioning" remains central – especially in the clinical context - since there is the question of when does conditioning exert protection among its various mechanisms.

The efficacy of postconditioning can readily be compared with ischemic preconditioning. This new, but promising strategy should start as early as possible after the onset of reperfusion to assure neuroprotection to open duration of this window would be important. As postconditioning may be easily clinical applicable, it has renders special attention. However, it was not know until present wheather postconditiong has any clinical relevance in the brain. Therefore, the present study give for the first time *experimental* evidence that postconditiong may be one therapeutic option to reach this goal in a selected patient subpopulation. The limitation of the effects of ischemic tolerance immediately after the onset of reperfusion after stroke in some animals speaks for the participation of oxygen radicals. In addition, the participation of other triggers relevant to reperfusion injury, such as complement-induced injuries, the cytokines (IL-6, IL-8, TNFα) and other inflammatory mediators (tissue factor, thrombin, protease activated receptors) should not be excluded from the menu of mechanisms to interrogate in pre- and postconditioning.

In addition, the present study introduce a modified, but new animal model to further examine the effect of postconditioning in the brain. It is the great advantage of this new animal model to have clinical relevance and may therefore be used to test clinical important question in an experimental model. The combination of this animal model with imaging methods opens the opportunity to visualize but also to monitor therapeutic effects in the brain.

Clinically, the most effective breakthrough in the treatment of cerebral ischemia has been the successful establishment of systemic thrombolysis. With the increasing knowledge about the dynamics of pathophysiological and molecular mechanisms leading to ischemia-related cell damage and about the presumed molecular targets of treatments counteracting these mechanisms, combinatorial treatment strategies based on thrombolysis and endogenous neuroprotection have to be developed. Ischemic tolerance in general and postconditioning in special – as demonstrated in the present study - seems to be a very strong candidate in serving a better understanding of the molecular mechanisms involved in neuroprotection as well as in improving therapeutic strategies for patients with stroke or other ischemia-related brain diseases. As demonstrated in the present study, molecular imaging techniques – like for example PET – may further help to visualize these molecular effects.

References

Abe H, Nowak TS (1996) Gene-expression and induced ischemic tolerance following brief insults. *Acta Neurobiol. Exp. (Warsz).* 56:3–8.

Akimitsu T, Gute DC, Korthuis RJ (1996). Ischemic preconditioning attenuates postischemic leukocyte adhesion and emigration. *Am. J. Physiol.* 40:H2052–H2059.

Aoki M, Abe K, Kawagoe J, et al. (1993) Acceleration of HSP70 and HSC70 heat shock gene expression following transient ischemia in the preconditioned gerbil hippocampus. *J. Cereb. Blood Flow Metab.* 13:781-8.

Araki T, Kato H, Kongure K. (1990) Neuronal damage and calcium accumulation following repeated brief cerebral ischemia in the gerbil. *Brain Res.* 528:114-22.

Arinowski J, Strong R, Grotta JC (1996) Combined neuroprotection and reperfusion therapy for stroke, -Effect of lubelzole and diaspirin cross-linked hemoglobulin in experimental focal ischemia. *Stroke* 27:1571-6.

Armstrong, S, Downey JM, Ganote CE (1994) Preconditioning of isolated rabbit cardiomyocyte induction by metabolic stress and blockade by the adenosine antagonist SPT and Calphostin C, and protein kinase C inhibitor. *Cardiovascul. Res.* 28:72-77.

Ashcroft FM (1988) Adenosine 5'-triphosphate-sensitive potassium channels. *Ann. Rev. Neurosci.* 11:97-118.

Astrup J, Siesjö BK, Symon L (1981) Threshold in cerebral ischamia – the ischemic penumbra. *Stroke* 12:723-5.

Barone FC, White RF, Spera PA, et al. (1998) Ischemic preconditioning and brain tolerance. *Stroke* 29:1937-51.

Baron JC, Frackowiak RSJ, herholz K (1989) Use of PET methods for measurements of cerebral energy metabolism and hemodynamics in cerebrovascular disease. *J. Cereb. Blood Flow Metab.* 9:723-742.

Baughman VL, Hoffman WE, Miletich DJ, et al (1988). Neurologic outcome in rats following incomplete cerebral ischemia during halothane, isoflurane or N_2O. *Anesthesiology.* 69: 192–198.

Baxter GF (2002) Role of adenosine in delayed preconditioning of myocardium. *Cardiovas. Res.* 55:483-494.

Baza N, Allan G (1998) *Platelet-activating factor and other bioactive lipids*. ed. Malden: Blackwell Science.

Belayev L, Ginsberg MD, Alonso OF, et al. (1996). Bilateral ischemic tolerance of rat hippocampus induced by prior unilateral transient focal ischemia: relationship to c-fos mRNA expression. *Neuroreport.* 8:55–59.

Bernardo NL, D'Angelo M, Okubo S, et al. (1999) Delayed ischemic preconditioning is mediated by opening of ATP-sensitive potassium channels in rabbit heart. *Am. J. Physiol.*, 276:H1323-H1330.

Bernaudin M, Nedelec AD, Divoux D, et al. (2002) Normobaric hypoxia induces tolerance to focal permanent cerebral ischemia in association with an increased expression of hypoxia-inducible factor-1 and its target genes, erythropoietin and VEGF, in the adult mouse brain. *J. Cereb. Blood Flow Metab.* 22:393-403.

Bergeron M, Gidday JM, Yu AY, et al (2000). Role of hypoxia-inducible factor-1 in hypoxia-induced ischemic tolerance in neonatal rat brain. *Ann. Neurol.* 48: 285–296.

Bestwick CS, Milne L (2000) Effects of beta-carotene on antioxidant enzyme activity, intracellular reactive oxygen and membrane integrity within post confluent Caco-2 intestinal cells. *Biochim. Biophys. Acta.* 1474:47-55

Bhardwaj A, Castro AFIII, Alkayed NJ, et al. (2001). Anesthetic choice of halothane versus propofol: impact on experimental perioperative stroke. *Stroke.* 32: 1920–1925.

Bjorkge JD, Jakymiw A, Fujita DJ (2000) Selected glimpses into the activation and function of Src kinase. *Oncogene* 19:5620-35.

Blanck TJ, Haile M, Xu F, et al (2000). Isoflurane pretreatment ameliorates postischemic neurologic dysfunction and preserves hippocampal Ca^{2+}/calmodulin-dependent protein kinase in a canine cardiac arrest model. *Anesthesiology.* 93: 1285–1293.

Blanco M, Lizasoain I, Sobrino T, et al. (2006) Ischemic preconditioning: a novel target for neuroprotective therapy. *Cerebrovasc Dis.* 21 Suppl 2:38-47.

Bordet R, Deplanque D, Maboudou P, et al (2000) Increase in endogenous brain superoxide dismutase as a potential mechanism of lipopolysaccaride-induced brain ischemic toleance. *J. Cereb. Blood Flow Metab.* 20:1190-6.

Brown MT, Cooper JA (1996) Regulation, substrates and functions of Src. *Biochim. Biophys. Acta.* 1287:121-49.

Bruno A, Levine SR, Frankel MR, et al. (2002) Admission glucose level and clinical outcomes in the NINDS rt-PA Stroke Trial. *Neurology* 59: 669–674.

Buchner K, Adamec E, Beermann ML, et al. (1999) Isoform-specific translocation of protein kinase C following glutamate administration in primary hippocampal neurons. *Molecular Brain Res.* 64:222-235.

Buisson A, Nicole O, Decogne F, et al. (1998) Up-regulation of a serine protease inhibitor in astrocytes mediates the neuroprotective activtiy of transforming growth factor beta1. *FASEB J.* 12:1683-91.

Busch HJ, Bushmann IR, Mies G, et al. (2003). Arteriogenesis in hypoperfused rat brain. *J. Cereb. Blood Flow Metab.* 23: 621–628.

Buschmann I, Schaper W (2000) The pathophysiology of the collateral circulation (arteriogenesis). *J. Pathol.* 190: 338–342.

Calabresi P, Centonze D, Bernardi G (2000) Cellular factors controlling neuronal vulnerability in the brain. A lesion from the striatum. *Neurology* 55:1249-55.

Carden DL, Granger DN (2000). Pathophysiology of ischaemia-reperfusion injury. *J. Pathol.* 190 :255 –266.

Chang J, Knowlton AA, Waser JS (2000) Expression of heat shock proteins in turtle and mammal hearts: relationship to anoxia tolerance. *Am. J. Physiol. Regul. Integr. Comp. Physiol.* 278:R209-14.

Chen J, Simon R (1997) Ischemic tolerance in the brain. *Neurology* 48:306-11.

Chiari PC, Bienengraeber MW, Pagel PS, et al. (2005) Isoflurane protects against myocardial infarction during early reperfusion by activation of physopatdylinositol-3-kinase signal transduciton: evidence for anesthetic-induced postconditioning in rabbits. *Anesthesiology* 102:102-9.

Chen D, Minami M, Hensahll DC, et al. (2003) Upregulation of mitochondrial base-excision repair capability within rat brain after brief ischemia. *J. Cereb. Blood Flow Metab.* 23:88-98.

Chen J, Simon R. (1997) .Ischemic tolerance in the brain. *Neurology*. 48:306-11.

Chen J, Graham S, Zhu R, et al. (1996) Stress proteins and tolerance to focal cerebral ischemia. *J. Cereb. Blood Flow Metab.* 16:566-77.

Chiari P, bouvet F, Piriou V (2005) Ansesthetic-induced myocardial preconditioning: fundamental basis and clinical implications. *Ann. Fr. Anesth Reanim.* 24:383-96.

Chiarugi A (2002) Characterization of the molecular events following impairment of NF-kappaB-driven transcription in neurons. *Brain Res. Mol Brain Res.* 109:179-88.

Ciechanover A, Orian A, Schwartz AL (2000) The ubiquitin-mediated proteolytic pathway: mode of action and clinical implications. *J. Cell Biochem. Suppl.* 34:40-51.

Chopp M, Li Y, Dereski MO, et al. (1992) Hypothermia reduces 72-kDA heatshock protein induction in rat brain after transient forebrain ischemia. *Stroke* 23:104-107.

Clark WM, Lutsep HL (1999). Medical treatment strategies: intravenous thrombolysis, neuronal protection, and anti-reperfusion injury agents. *Neuroimaging Clin. N Am.* 9 :465 –473.

Cohen MV, Baines CP, Downey JM (2000) Ischemic preconditioning: from adenosine receptor to K_{ATP} channel. *Annu. Rev. Physiol.* 62:79-109.

Cole WC (1993) ATP-sensitive K^+ channels in cardiac ischemia: an endogenous mechanism for protection of the heart, *Cardiovasc. Drugs Ther.* 7:527-537.

Corbett D, Crooks P (1997) Ischemic preconditioning: a long term survival study using behavorial and histological endpoints. *Brain Res.* 1997; 760:129-36.

Couglin SR (2000) Thrombin signalling and proteas-activated receptors. *Nature* 407:258-64.

Coyle P, Heistad DD (1991) Development of collaterals in the cerebral circulation. *Blood Vessels.* 28: 183–189.

Coyle P (1984). Diameter and length changes in cerebral collaterals after middle cerebral artery occlusion in the young rat. *Anat. Rec.* 210:357–364.

Currie W, Ellison JA, white RF, et al. (2000) Benign focal ischemic preconditioning induces neuronal HSP70 and prolonged astrogliosisy with expression of HSP27. *Brain Res.* 863:169-81.

Daffertshofer M, Mielke O, Pullwitt A, et al. (2004) Transient ischemic attacks are more than "ministrokes". *Stroke.* 35:2453-8.

Dana A, Skarli M, Papakrivopoulou J, et al. (2000) Adenosine A(1) receptor induced delayed preconditioning in rabbits: induction of p38 mitogen-activated protein kinase activation and Hsp27 phosphorylation via a tyrosine kinase- and protein kinase C-dependent mechanism. *Circ. Res.* 86:989-997.

Danton GH, Dietrich WD (2004) The search for neuroprotective strategies in stroke. *Am. J. Neuroradiol.* 25:181-94.

Darling CE, Jiang R, Maynard M, et al. (2005) Postconditioning via stuttering reperfusion limits myocardial ischemia-reperfusion limits myocardial infarct size in rabbit hearts: role of ERK1/2. *Am. J. Physiol. Heart Circ. Physiol.* 289:H1618-26.

Das DK, Engelman RM, Maulik N (1999) Oxygen free radical signaling in ischemic preconditioning, *Ann. N. Y. Acad. Sci.*, 874:49-65.

Das R, Mahabeleshwar GH, Kundu GC (2003) Osteopontin stimulates cell motility and nuclear factor kappaB-mediated secretion of urokinase type plasminogen activator through phosphatidylinositol 3-kinase/Akt signaling pathways in breast cancer cells. *J. Biol. Chem.* 278:28593-606.

Daval JL, Nicolas F (1994) Opposite effects of cyclohexyladenosine and theophylline on hypoxic damage in cultured neurons, *Neurosci. Lett.*, 175:114-116.

Dawn B, Xuan YT, Qiu Y, et al. (1999) Bifunctional role of protein tyrosine kinases in late preconditioning against myocardial stunning in conscious rabbits. *Circ. Res.* 85:1154-1163.

Dawn B, Bolli R (2002) Role of nitric oxide in myocardial preconditioning. *Ann. N. Y. Acad. Sci.* 962:18-41.

Dawn B, Takano H, Tang XL, et al. (2002b) Role of Src protein tyrosine kinases in late preconditioning against myocardial infarction. *Am. J. Physiol. Heart Circ. Physiol.* 283:H549-56.

Dawson TM (2002) Preconditioningn-mediated heurportection through erythropoietin? Lancet 359:96-97.

DeGracia DJ, Kumar R, Owen CR, et al. (2002) Molecular pathways of protein synthesis inhibition during brain reperfusion: implicaitons for neuronal survival or death. *J. Cereb. Blood Flow Metab.* 22:393-403.

del Zoppo GJ, Mabuchi T (2003) Cerebral microvessel responses to focal ischemia. *J. Cereb. Blood Flow Metab.* 23: 879–894.

Diaz RJ, Wilson GJ (2004) Modifying the first minute of reperfusion: potential for myocardial salvage. *Cardiovasc Res.* 62:4-6.

Di Capua N, Sperling O, Zoref-Shani E (2003) Protein kinase C-ε is involved in the adenosine-activated signal transduction pathway conferring protection against ischemia-reperfusion injury in primary rat neuronal cultures, *J. Neurochem.* 84:409-412.

Digicaylioglu M, Lipton SA (2001) Erythropoietin-mediated neuroprotection involves cross-talk between Jak" and NF-κB signaling cascades. *Nature* 412:614-47.

Dirnagl U, Iadecola C, Moskowitz MA (1999) Pathobiology of ischemic stroke: an integrated view. *Trends Neurosci* 22:391-7.

Dirnagl U, Simon RP, Hallenbeck JM, et al. (1993) The pharmacology of ATP-sensitive potassium channels. *Ann. Rev. Pharmacol. Toxicol.* 33:597-637.

Dowden J, Corbett D. (1999) Ischemic preconditioning in 18- to 20-month-old gerbils: long-term survival with functional outcome measures. *Stroke*. 30:1240-6.

Droge W (2002) Free radicals in the physiological control of cell function. *Physiol Rev*. 82, 47-95.

Du C, Hu R, Csernansky CA, et al. (1996). Very delayed infarction after mild focal cerebral ischemia: a role for apoptosis? *J. Cereb. Blood Flow Metab.* 16: 195–201.

Edwards AD, Yue X, Squier MV, et al. (1995) Specific inhibition of apoptosis after cerebral hypoxia-ischaemia by moderate post-insult hypothermia. *Biochem. Biophys. Res. Commun.* 217: 1193–1199.

Eguchi Y, Shimizu S, Tsujimoto Y (1997) Intracellular ATP levels determine cell death fate by apoptosis or necrosis. *Cancer Res*. 1997; 57:1835-40.

Ehrenreich H. (2004) Medicine. A boost for translational neuroscience. *Science* 305:184-185.

Ehrenreich H, Hasselblatt M, Dembowski C et al. (2002) Erythropoietin therapy for acute stroke in both safe and beneficial. *Mol. Med.* 8:495-505.

Emerich DF, Dean RL III, Bartus RT (2002) The role of leukocytes following cerebral ischemia: pathogenic variable or bystander reaction to emerging infarct? *Exp. Neurol.* 173: 168–181.

Erecinska M, Thoresen M, Silver IA. (2003) Effects of hypothermia on energy metabolism in mammalian central nervous system. *J. Cereb. Blood Flow Metab.* 23:513 –530.

Eriksson L, Holte S, Bohm C, et al. (1988) Automated blood sampling systems for positron emission tomography. *IEET Trans Nucl. Sci.* 35:703-704.

Ettaiche M, Heurteaux C, Blondeau N, et al. (2001) ATP-sensitive potassium channels (K(ATP)) in retina: a key role for delayed ischemic tolerance. *Brain Res*. 890:118-29.

Feng J, Luccinetti E, Ahuja P et al. Isoflurane postconditioning prevents opening of the mitochondrial permeability transition pore through inhibition of glycogen synthase kianse 3beta. *Anesthesiology* 103:987-95.

Ferriero DM. (2005) Protecting neurons. *Epilepsia*. 46 Suppl 7:45-51.

Fisher M, Ratan R (2003) New perspectives on developing acute stroke therapy. *Ann. Neurol.* 53:10-20.

Fisher M, Takano K. (1995) The penumbra, therapeutic time window and acute ischaemic stroke. *Baillieres Clin. Neurol.* 4:279-95.

Forbes RA, Steenbergen C, Murphy E (2001) Diazoxide-induced cardioprotection requires signaling through a redox-sensitive mechanism, *Circ. Res*. 88:802-9.

Fredholm BB,.Arslan G, Halldner L, et al. (2000) Structure and function of adenosine receptors and their genes, *Naunyn Schmiedebergs Arch. Pharmacol.* 362:364-74.

Freeman BA, Crapo JD (1982) Biology of disease: free radials and tissue injury. *Lab. Invest* 47:412-26.

Frerichs KU, Deckert M, Kempski O, et al. (1994) Local cerebral blood flow during hibernation, a model of natural tolerance to "cerebral ischemia". *J. Cereb. Blood Flow. Metab.* 14:193-205.

Freund S, Ungerer M, Lohse MJ (1994) A1 adenosine receptors expressed in CHO-cells couple to adenylyl cyclase and to phospholipase C, *Naunyn Schmiedebergs Arch. Pharmacol.* 350:49-56.

Fryer RM, Schultz JEJ, Hsu AK, et al. (1999) Importance of PKC and tyrosine kinase in single or multiple cycles of preconditioning in rat hearts. *Am. J. Physiol. Heart Circ. Physiol.* 276:H1229-H1235.

Fryer RM, Hsu AK, Eells JT, et al. (1999) Opioid-induced second window of cardioprotection; potential role of K_{ATP} channels, *Circ. Res.* 84:846-851.

Furuta S, Ohta S, Hatakeyama T, et al. (1993) Recovery of protein synthesis in tolerance-induced hippocampal CA1 neurons after transient forebrain ischemia. *Acta Neuropathol. (Berl)* 86:329-36.

Garlid KD, Dos Santos P, Xie ZJ, et al. (2003) Mitochondrial potassium transport: the role of the mitochondrial ATP-sensitive K(+) channel in cardiac function and cardioprotection. *Biochim. Biophys. Acta.* 1606:1-21.

Geddes JW, Pettigrew LC, Holtz ML, et al. (1996) Permanent focal and transient global cerebral ischemia increase glial and neuronal expression of heme oxygenase-1 but not heme oxygenase-2, protein in rat brain. *Neuroscience Lett.* 210:205-8.

Gentile NT, Spatz M, Brenner M, et al. (1996) Decreased calcium accumulation in isolated nerve endings during hibernation in ground squirrels. *Neurohem. Res.* 21:947-54.

Gerasimov VD, Artemenko DP, Krishtal OA (2001) Preconditioning by motor activity protects rat hippocampal CA1 neurons against prolonged ischemia. *Brain Res.* 888:326-9.

Gho BC, Schoemaker RG, van den Doel MA, et al. (1996) Myocardial protection by brief ischemia in noncardiac tissue. *Circulation* 94:2193-200.

Gidday JM. (2006) Cerebral preconditioning and ischaemic tolerance. *Nat. Rev. Neurosci.* 7:437-48.

Gidday JM, Fitzgibbons JC, Shah AR, et al. (1994) Neuroprotection from ischemic brain injury by hypoxic preconditioning in the neonatal rat. *Neurosci. Lett.* 168:221-224.

Gjedde A, Wienhard K, Heiss WD, et al. (1985) Comparative regional analysis of 2-fluorodeoxyglucose and methylglucose uptake in brain of four stroke patients. With special reference to the regional estimation of the lumped constant. *J. Cereb. Blood Flow Metab.* 5: 137–168.

Glazier SS, O'Rourke DM, Graham DI, et la. (1994) Induction of ischemic tolerance following biref local ischemia in rat brain. *J. Cereb. Blood Flow Metab.* 14:545-53.

Gladstone DJ, Black SE, Hakim AM (2002) Toward wisdom from failure: lessons from neuroprotective stroke trials and new therapeutic directions. *Stroke* 33 :2123 –2136.

Glover JR, Lindquist S (1998) HSP 104, HSP 70, and HSP 40: A novel chaperone system that rescues previousyl aggregated proteins. *Cell* 94:73-82.

Goldberg MP, Monyer H, Eeiss JH, et al. (1988) Adenosine reduces cortical neuronal injury induced by oxygen or glucose deprivation in vitro, *Neurosci Lett* 89:323-327.

Goodal AR, Turner NA, Walker JH, et al. (1997) Activation of protein kinase C-alpha and translocation of the myristoylated alanine-rich C-kinase substrate correlate with phorbol ester-enhanced noradrenaline release from SH-SY5Y human neuroblastoma cells, *J. Neurochem.* 68:392-401.

Goodman Y, burce AJ, Cheng B, et al. (1996) Ceramide protects hippocampal neurons against excitotoxic and oxidative insults, and amyloid beta-peptide toxicity. *J. Neurochem.* 66:1836-44.

Golden WC, Brambrink Am, Traystman RJ, et al. Failure to sustain recovery of Na,K-ATPase function is a possible mechanism for striatal neurodegeneration in hypoxic-ischemic newborn piglets. *Brain Res. Mol. Brain Res.* 88:94-102.

Gonzalez-Zulueta M, Feldman AB, Klesse LJ, et al. (2000) Requrirement for nitrico xoide activation of p21ras7 extracellular regulated kinase in neuronal ischemic preconditioning. *PNAS* 97:436-441.

Grabb MC, Choi DW (1999) Ischemic tolerance in murine cortical cell culture: critical role for NMDA receptors. *J. Neurosci.* 19:1657-62.

Graf R, Sanada Y, Dohmen C, Schaller B, et al. (2004) Early hemicraniectomy may rescue tissue at risk after middle cerebral artery occlusion in cats. A sequential PET study. *Stroke* 35:E247.

Graf R, Wienhard K, Löttgen J, et al. (1996) Transient focal ischemia in cats: dynamics of blood flow and metabolism determined by PET in Krieglsten J (ed): Pharmacology of cerebral ischemia. Wissenschaftliche Verlagsgesellschaft mBH Stuttgart, pp 315-25.

Graf R, Kataoka K, Rosner G, et al. (1986) Cortical differentiation in cat focal ischemia: disturbance and recovery of sensory functions in corticalareas with different degrees of cerebral blood flow reduction. *J. Cereb. Blood Flow Metab.* 6: 566-573.

Graham SH, et al. (2002) Expression of the proto-oncogene bcl-2 is increased in the rat bain following kainite-induced seizures. *Restor. Neurol. Neurosci.* 9:243-50.

Grotta JC (1999). Acute stroke therapy at the millennium: consummating the marriage between the laboratory and bedside: the Feinberg lecture. *Stroke* 30:1722 –1728.

Grover GJ (1996) Role of the ATP-sensitive potassium channel in ischaemic preconditioning, In Marber MS and Yellon DM (Eds.) *Ischemia: preconditioning and adaptation*, BIOS Scientific Publishers Ltd, Oxford, pp. 35-58.

Gumina RJ, Gross GJ (1999) If ischemic preconditioning is the gold standard, has a platinum standard of cardioprotection arrived? Comparison with NHE inhibition. *J. Thromb. Thrombolysis* 8:39-44.

Guo Y, Jones WK, Xuan YT, et al. (1999) The late phase of ischemic preconditioning is abrogated by targeted disruption of the inducible NO synthase gene. *Proc. Natl. Acad. Sci. USA.* 96: 11507–11512.

Guo Z, Cooper LF (2000) An N-terminal 33-amino-acid-deletion variant of hsp 25 retains oligomerization and functional properties. *Biochem. Biophys. Res. Commun.* 270:183-9.

Hacke W, Kaste M, Fieschi C, et al. (1998) Randomised double-blind placebo-controlled trial of thrombolytic therapy with intravenous alteplase in acute ischaemic stroke (ECASS II): Second European-Australasian Acute Stroke Study Investigators. *Lancet* 352 :1245 – 1251.

Haddad GG, Ma E (2001) Neuronal tolerance to O2 deprivation in Drosphila: novel approaches using genetic models. *Neuroscientist* 7:538-50.

Haddad GG, Jiang C (1994) Mechanisms of neuronal survival during hypoxia: ATP-sensitive K^+ channels, *Bio. Neonate*, 65:160-165.

Halkos ME; Kerendi F, Corvera JS, et al. (2004) Myocardial protection with postconditioning is not enhanced by ischemic preconditioning. *Ann. Thorac. Surg.* 78:961-9.

Hamaya Y, Takeda T, Dohi S, et al. (2000). The effects of pentobarbital, isoflurane and propofol on immediate-early gene expression in the vital organs of the rat. *Anesth. Analg.* 90: 1177–1183.

Hartl FU (1996) Molecular chaperons in cellular protein folding. *Nature* 381:571-9.

Hattori R, Otani H, Uchiyama T, et al. (2001) Src tyrosine kinase is the trigger but not the mediator of ischemic preconditioning. *Am. J. Physiol. Heart Circ. Physiol.* 281:H1066-74.

Hawaleshak A, Jacobsohn E (1998) Ischemic preconditioning: mechanism and potential clinical applications (Review). *Can. J. Anaesth* 45:670-82.

Heiss WD, Thiel A, Grond M, et al. (1999) Which targets are relevant for therapy of acute ischemic stroke? *Stroke* 30:1486-89.

Heiss WD, Graf R, Löttgen J, et al. (1997) Repeated positron emission tomographic studies in transient middle cerebral artery occlusion in cats: Residual perfusion and efficacy of postischemic reperfusion. *J. Cereb. Blood Flow Metab.* 17:388-400.

Heiss WD, Grond M, Thiel A, et al. (1997) Ischemic brain tisue salvaged from infarction with alteplase. *Lancet* 349:1599-600.

Heiss WD, Graf R, Wienhard K, et al. (1994) Dynamic penumbra demonstrated by sequential multitracer PET after middle cerebral artery occlusion in cats. *J. Cereb. Blood Flow Metab.* 14:892-902.

Heiss WD (1992) Experimenta evidence for ischemic thresholds and functional recovery. *Stroke* 23:1668-72.

Heiss WD, Rosner G (1983) functional recovery of cortical neurons as related to degree and duration of ischemia. *Ann. Neurol.* 14:294-301.

Heiss WD, Hayakawa T, Walz AG (1976) Cortical neuronal function during ischemia. *Arch. Neurol.* 33:813-20.

Herbert DA, Mitchell RA (1971) Blood gas tensions and acidic balance in awake cats. *J. Appl. Physiol.* 30:434-436.

Herscovitch P, Markham J, Raichle ME (1983) Brain blood flow measured with intravenous H2-15O. I: theory and error analysis. *J. Nucl. Med.* 24:782-789.

Heurteaux C, Lauritzen I, Widmann C, et al. (1995) Essential role of adenosine, adenosine A1 receptors, and ATP-sensitive K+ channels in cerebral ischemic preconditioning. *Proc. Natl. Acad. Sci. USA* 92:4666-4670.

Heurteaux C, Bertaina V, Widmann C, et al. (1993) K^+ channel openers prevent global ischemia-induced expression of c-*fos*, c-*jun*, heat shock protein, and amyloid β-protein precursor genes and neuronal death in rat hippocampus, *Proc. Natl. Acad. Sci., USA,* 90:9431-9435.

Heusch G (2004) Postconditioning: old win in a new bottle? *J. Am. Coll Cardiol.* 44:1111-2.

Higashida RT, Furlan AJ, Roberts H, et al. .(2003) Trial design and reporting standards for intra-arterial cerebral thrombolysis for acute ischemic stroke. *Stroke.* 34:e109-37.

Hirakawa T, Rokutan K, Nikawa T, et al. (1996) Geranylgeranyl acetone unduces heat shock proteins in cultured guined pig gastric mucosal cells and rat gastric mucosa. *Gastroenterology* 111:345-357.

Hochachka PW, Lutz PL (2001) Mechanism, origin, and evolution of anoxia tolerance in animals. *Comp. Biochem. Physiol. Biochem. Mol. Bio.* 130:435-459.

Hossmann KA (1994) Viability thresholds and the penumbra of focal ischemia. *Ann. Neurol.* 36: 557–565.

Hsu CY, An G, Liu JS, et al. (1993). Expression of immediate early gene and growth factor mRNAs in a focal cerebral ischemia model in the rat. *Stroke.* (suppl I);24:I-78–I-81.

Hua Y, Xi G, Keep RF, et al. (2000) Plaminogen activator inhibitor-1 induction after experimental intracerebral hemorrhage. *Stroke* 31:794-5.

Huang KP, Huang FL, Nakabayashi H, et al. (1988) Biochemical characterization of rat brain protein kinase C isozymes, *J. Biol. Chem.*, 263:14839-14845.

Huber R, Kasischke K, Ludolph AC, et al. (1999) Increase of cellular hypoxic tolerance by erythromycin and other antibiotics. *Neuroreport* 10:1543-46.

Igelmund P, et al. Hibernation and hippocampal transmission. In: *Adaptions to the cold: Tennth International Hiberation Symposiim Armidale.* In: Geiser F, et al. (eds). pp, 159.165

Inagaki K, Hahn HS, Dorn GW 2nd, et al. (2003) Additive protection of the ischemic heart ex vivo by combined treatment with delta-protein kinase C inhibitor and epsilon-protein kinase C activator, *Circulation* 108:869-75.

Iwasa Y, Hosey MM (1984) Phosphorylation of cardiac sarcolemma proteins by the calcuim-activated phospholipid-dependent protein kinase, *J. Biol. Chem.*, 259:534-540.

Jain KK (2000). Neuroprotection in cerebrovascular disease. *Expert Opin. Investig Drugs* 9:695 –711.

Jinag Y, Zhu D, Okagaki P , et al. (2003) N-methyl-D-aspartate and Trk B receptor activation in cerebellar granule cells. An in vitro model of preconditioning to stimulate intrinsic survival pathways in neurons. *Ann. NY Acad. Sci.* 993:134-45.

Jiang Y, Wu J, Hua Y, et al. (2002) Thrombin-receptor activation and thrombin-induced brain tolerance. *J. Cereb. Blood Flow Metab.* 22:404-10.

Jones NM, Bergeron M (2001) Hypoxic preconditioningn in capable of inducing mitochondrial tolerance in the rat brain. *J. Cereb. Blood Flow Metab.* 21:1105-14.

Johnson JA, Gray MO, Chen CH, et al. (1996) A protein kinase C translocation inhibitor as an isozyme-selective antagonist of cardiac function. *J. Biol. Chem.*, 271:24962-24966.

Kaeffer N, Richard V, Francois A, et al. (1996) Preconditioning prevents chronic reperfusion-induced coronary endothelial dysfunction. *Am. J. Physiol.* 271:H842–H849.

Kanemitsu H, Nakagomi T, Tamura A, et al (2002). Differences in the extent of primary ischemic damage between middle cerebral artery coagulation and intraluminal occlusion models. *J. Cereb. Blood Flow Metab.* 22: 1196–1204.

Kapinya K, Penzel R, Sommer C, et al. (2000). Temporary changes of the AP-1 transcription factor binding activity in the gerbil hippocampus after transient global ischemia, and ischemic tolerance induction. *Brain Res.* 872: 282–293.

Kasischke K, Carpenter DO, Riepe MW (1997) Chemical preconditioning can be induced repeatedly. *Soc. Neurosci. Abstr.* 2183.

Kasischke K, Huber R, Li H, et al. (1999) Primary hypoxic tolerance and chemical preconditioning during estrus cycle in mice. *Stroke* 30:1256-62.

Kassem-Moussa H, Graffagnino C (2002). Nonocclusion and spontaneous recanalization rates in acute ischemic stroke: a review of cerebral angiography studies. *Arch. Neurol.* 59: 1870–1873.

Kato H, Liu Y, Araki T, et al. (1991) Temporal profile of the effects of pretreatment with brief cerebral ischemia on the neuronal damage following secondary ischemic insult in the gerbil: cumulative damage and protective effects, *Brain Res*. 553:238-242.

Kato H, Liu Y, Kogure K, et al. (1994a) Induction of 27-kDa heat shock protein following cerebral ischemia in a rat model of ischemic tolerance, *Brain Res*. 634:235-244.

Kato H, Kogure K, Liu Y, et al. (1994b) Induction of NADPH-diaphorase activity in the hippocampus in rat model of cerebral ischemia and ischemic tolerance, *Brain Res*. 652:71-75.

Kato H, Liu Y, Arki T, et al. (1992) Mk-801, but not aniosmycin, inhibits the induction of tolerance to ischemia in the gerbil hippocampus. *Neurosci Lett*. 139:118-21.

Kerendi F, Kin H, Halkos ME, et al. (2005) Remote postconditioning. Brief renal ischemia and reperfsuion applied befreo coronrary artery reperfusion reduces myocardial infarct size via endogenous activation of adenosine receptors. *Basic Res. Cardiol* 100:404-12.

Kihara T, Shimohama S, Sawada H, et al. (2001) alpha 7 nicotinic receptor transduces signals to phosphatidylinositol 3-kinase to block A beta-amyloid-induced neurotoxicity. *J. Biol. Chem*. 276:13541-6.

Kim WK, Choi YB, Rayudu PV, et al. (1999). Attenuation of NMDA receptor activity and neurotoxicity by nitroxyl anion, NO-. *Neuron*. 24:461–469.

Kapinya KJ, Lowl D, Futterer C, et al. (2002) Tolerance against ischemic neuronal injury can be induced by volatile anesthetics and is inducible NO synthase dependent. *Stroke*. 33:1889-98.

Kato H, Liu Y, Araki T, et al. (1991) Temporal profile of the effects of pretreatment with brief cerebral ischemia on the neuronal damage following secondary ischemic insult in the gerbil: cumulative damage and protective effects. *Brain Res*. 553:238-42.

Kharbanda RK, Peters M, Walton B, et al. (2001) Ischemic preconditioning prevents endothelial injury and systemic neutrophil activation during ischemia-reperfusion in humans in vivo. *Circulation* 103:1624-30.

Kaspekov L, Shamloo M, Victorov I, et al. (1998) Sublethal in vitor glucose-oxygen deprivation protects cultured hippocampal neurons against a subsequent severe insult. *Neuroreport* 9:1273-6.

Kehrer JP (1993) Free radicals as mediators of tissue injury and disease. *Crit. Rev. Toxicol*. 23:21-48.

Kin H, Zatta AJ, Jiang R, et al. (2005) Activation of opiod receptors mediates the infarct size reduction by postconditioning. *J. Mol. Cell Cardiol*. 38:827 (Abstract).

Kin H, Zhao ZQ, Sun HY, et al. (2004) Postconditioning attenuates myocardial ischemia-reperfusion injury by inhibiting events in the early minutes of reperfusion. *Cardiovasc. Res*. 62:74-85.

Kirino T. (2002) Ischemic tolerance. *J. Cereb. Blood Flow Metab*. 22:1283-96.

Kirino T, Tsujita Y, Tamura A (1991) Induced tolerance to ischemia in gerbil hippocampal neurons, *J. Cereb. Blood Flow Metab*. 11:299-307.

Kitagawa K, Yagita Y, Sasaki T, et al. (2005) Chronic mild reduction of cerebral perfusion pressure induces ischemic tolerance in focal cerebral ischemia. *Stroke*. 36:2270-4.

Kitigawa K, Matsumoto M, Kuwabara K, et al. (1991) Ischemic tolerance phenomenon in various brain regions. *Brain Res*. 561:203-1.

Kitigawa K, Matsumoto M, Tagaya M, et al. (1990) Ischemic tolerance phenomenon found in the brain. *Brain Res*.528:21-4.

Kleihues P, Hosmann KA (1971) Protein synthesis in the cat brain after prolonged cerebral ischemia. *Brain Res* 35:409-18.

Kobayashi S, Harris VA, Welsh FA (1995) Spreading depression induces tolerance of cortical neurons to ischemia in rat brain. *J. Cereb. Blood Flow Metab.* 15:721–727.

Kraig RP, Dong LM, Thisted R, et al. (1991). Spreading depression increases immunohistochemical staining of glial fibrillary acidic protein. *J. Neurosci.* 11:2187–2198.

Krieglstein J, Rischke R (1991) Vinpocetin increases the neuroprotective effect of adenosine in vitro. *Europ. J. Pharmacol.*, 205:7-10.

Kristian, T, Siesjö BK (1998) Calcium in ischemic cell death. *Stroke* 29:705-18.

Kukreja RC (2002) NFkappaB activation during ischemia/reperfusion in heart: friend or foe? *J. Mol. Cell Cardiol.* 34:1301-4.

Kuzuya T, Hoshida S, Yamashita N, et al. (1993) Delayed effects of sublethal ischemia on the equisition of tolerance to ischemia, *Circ. Res.*, 72:1293-1299.

Landau E, Tirsoh R, Pinson A, et al. (2000) Protection of thrombin receptor expression under hypoxia. *J. Biol. Chem.* 275:2281-7.

Lauritzen I, De Weille JR, Lazdunski M (1997) The potassium channel opener (-)-cromakalim prevents glutamate-induced cell death in hippocampal neurons, *J. Neurochem.* 69:1570-1579.

Lee JM, Grabb MC, Zipfel GJ, et al. (2000) Brain tissue responses to ischemia. *J. Clin. Investigat.* 106:723-73.

Leist M, Single B, Castoldy AF, et al. (1997) Intracellular adenosine triphosphate concentration: a switch in the decision between apoptosis and necrosis. *J. Exp. Med.* 185:1481-6.

Lennon SV, Martin SJ, Cotter TG (1991) Dose dependent induction of apoptosis in human tumor cell lines by widely diverging stimuli. *Cell Prolif.* 24:203-14.

Leesar MA, Stoddard MF, Dawn B, et al. (2001). Delayed preconditioning-mimetic action of nitroglycerin in patients undergoing coronary angioplasty. *Circulation.* 103: 2935–2941.

Liebeskind DS (2003). Collateral circulation. *Stroke.* 34:2279–2284.

Light PE, Sabir AA, Allen BG, et al. (1996) Protein kinase C-induced changes in the stoichiometry of ATP binding activate cardiac ATP-sensitive K^+ channels. A possible mechanistic link to ischemic preconditioning, *Circ. Res.* 79:399-406.

Lin B, Globus MY, Dietrich WD, et al. (1992) Differing neurochemical and morphological sequelae of global ischemia: comparison of single- and multiple-insult paradigms. *J. Neurochem.* 59:2213-23.

Lipton P (1999). Ischemic cell death in brain neurons. *Physiol. Rev.* 79:1431–1568.

Liu D, Lu C, Wan R, et al. (2002) Activation of mitochondrial ATP-dependende potassium channels protects neurons against ischemia-induced death by a mechanism involving suppression of Bax translocation and cytochrom c release. *J. Cereb. Blood Flow Metab.* 21:1105-14.

Liu J, Ginis I, Saptz M, et al. (2000) Hypoxic preconditioningn protects cultured neurons against hypoxic stress via TNF-alpha and ceramide. *Am. J. Physiol. Cell Physiol.* 278:C144-53.

Liu Y, Kato H, Kato N, et al. (1992) Protection of rat hippocampus against ischemic neuronal damage by pretreatment with sublethal ischemia, *Brain Res,* 586:121-124.

Liu Y, Kato H, Nakat N, et al. (1993) Temporal profile of heat shock protein 70 synthesis in ischemic tolerance induced by preconditioning ischemia in rat hippocampus, *Neuroscience* 56:921-927.

Liu Y, Gao WD, O'Rourke B., et al. (1996) Synergistic modulation of ATP-sensitive K^+ currents by protein kinase C and adenosine. Implications for ischemic preconditioning, *Circ. Res.* 78:443-454.

Lo EH, Dalkara T, Moskowitz MA (2003) Mechsnisms, challenges and opportunities in stroke. *Nat. Rev. Neurosci.* 4:399-415.

Lovett JK, Dennis MS, Sandercock PA, et al. (2003) Very early risk of stroke after a first transient ischemic attack. *Stroke*. 34: e138–e140.

Luccinetti E, da Silva R, Pasch T, et al. (2005) Anaesthetic preconditioning but not postconditioning prevents early activation of the deleterious cardiac remodeling programme: evidence of opposing genomic responses in cardioprotection by pre- and postconditioning. *Br. J. Anaesth.* 95:140-52.

Lutz PL, Nilsson GE (1997) Contrasting strategies for anoxic brain survival-glycolysis up or down. *J. Exp. Biol.* 200:411-9.

Ma YC, Huang XY (2002) Novel regulation and function of Src tyrosine kinase. *Cell. Mol. Life Sci.* 59:456-62.

Marota JJ, Crosby G, Uhl GR (1992) Selective effects of pentobarbital and halothane on c-fos and jun-B gene expression in rat brain. *Anesthesiology.* 77: 365–371.

Marshall JW, Duffin KJ, Green AR, et al. (2001). NXY-059, a free radical–trapping agent, substantially lessens the functional disability resulting from cerebral ischemia in a primate species. *Stroke* 32: 190–198.

Matsumishma K, Hakim AM (1995) Transient forebrain ischemia protects agianst subsequent focal cerebral ischemia without changing cerebral perfusion. *Stroke* 26:1047-52.

Matsushima K, Hogan MJ, Hakim AM (1996). Cortical spreading depression protects against subsequent focal cerebral ischemia in rats. *J. Cereb. Blood Flow Metab.* 16:221–226.

Matsushima K, Hakim AM (1995) Transient forebrain ischemia protects against subsequent focal cerebral ischemia without changing cerebral perfusion. *Stroke* 26:1047-52.

Miyashita K, Abe H, Nakajima T, et al. (1994) Induction of ischemic tolerance in gerbil hippocampus by pre-treatment with focal ischemia. *Neuroreport* 14:945-8.

Miettinen S, Roivainen R, Keinanen R, et al. (1996) Specific induction of protein kinase C delta subspecies after transient middle cerebral artery occlusion in the rat brain: inhibition by MK-801, *J. Neurosci.* 16:6236-45.

Mintun MA; Raichle ME; Martin WRW (1984) Brain oxygen utilization measured with O15 radiotracers and positron emission tomography. *J. Nucl. Med.* 25:177-187.

Miura Y, Grocott HP, Bart RD, et al. (1998). Differential effects of anesthetic agents on outcome from near-complete but not incomplete global ischemia in the rat. *Anesthesiology.* 89: 391–400.

Moncayo J, de Freitas GR, Bogousslavsky J, et al. (2000) Do transient ischemic attacks have a neuroprotective effect? *Neurology*. 54:2089-94.

Moro MA; Almeida A, Bolanos JP, et al. (2005) Mitochondiral respiratory chain and free radical generation in stroke. *Free Radic. Biol. Med.* 39:1291-304.

Munshi R, Pang IH, Sternweis PC, et al. (1991) A1 adenosine receptors of bovine brain couple to guanine nucleotide-binding proteins Gi1, Gi2, and Go. *J. Biol. Chem.* 266:22285-9.

Murphy, K.P.S.J. and Greenfield, S.A. (1991) ATP-sensitive potassium channels counteract anoxia in neurons of the substantia nigra, *Exp. Brain Res.* 84:355-358.

Murry CE, Jennings RB, Reimer KA (1986) Preconditioning with ischemia: A delay of lethal cell injury in ischemic myocardium, *Circulation*, 74:1124-1136.

Nagai N, DeMol M, Lijnen HR, et al. (1999) Role of plasminogen system components in focal cerebral ischemic infarction: a gene targeting and gene transfer study in mice. *Circulation* 99:2440-4.

Nakagomi T, Kirino T, Kanemitsu H, et al. (1993) Early recovery of protein synthesis following ischemia in hippocampal neurons with induced tolerance in the gerbil. *Acta Neuropathol.* 86:10-5.

Nakano A, Cohen MV, Downey JM (2000) Ischemic preconditioning: from basic mechanisms to clinical applications, *Pharmacol. Ther.* 86:263-75.

Nakata N, Kato H, Kongrue K (1993) Inhibition of ischemic tolerance in the gerbil hippocampus by quercetin and anti-heat shock protein-70antibody. *Neuroreport* 4:695-8.

Nakayama H, Dietrich WD, Watson BD, et al (1988). Photothrombotic occlusion of rat middle cerebral artery: histopathological and hemodynamic sequelae of acute recanalization. *J. Cereb. Blood Flow Metab.* 8 :357 –366.

Nawashiro H, Tasaki K, Ruetzler CA, et al. TNF-alpha pre-treatment induces protective effects against focal cerebral ischemia in mice. *J. Cereb. Blood Flow Metab.* 17:483-90.

Nishi S, Taki W, Uemura Y, et al. (1993) Ischemic tolerance due to the induction of HSP70 in a rat ischemic recirculation model, *Brain Res.*, 615:281-288.

Nishizuka Y (1986) Studies and perspectives of protein kinase C, *Science*, 233:305-312.

Nishizuka Y (1989) The Albert Lasker Medical Awards: the family of protein kinase C for signal transduction, *J. Am. Med. Assoc.*, 262:1826-1833.

Ohta K, Graf R, Rosner G, et al. (1997) Profiles of cortical tissue depolarization in cat focal cerebral ischemia in relation to calcium ion homeostasis and nitric oxide production. *J. Cereb. Blood Flow Metab* 17:1170-1181.

Ohtsuki T, ruetzler CA, Tatsaki K, et al. (1996) Interleukin-1 mediates induction of tolerance to global ischemia in gerbil hippocampal CA1 neurons. *J. Cereb. Blood Flow Metab.* 16:1137-42.

Ohtsuki T, Matsumoto M, Kitagawa K, et al. (1993). Induced resistance and susceptibility to cerebral ischemia in gerbil hippocampal neurons by prolonged but mild hypoperfusion. *Brain Res.* 614: 279–284.

Ohtsuki T, Matsumoto M, Kuwabara K, et al. (1992) Influence of oxidative stress on induced tolerance to ischemia in gerbil hippocampal neurons. *Brain Res.* 599:246-52.

Okubo S, Bernardo NL, Elliott GT, et al. (2000) Tyrosine kinase signaling in action potential shortening and expression of HSP72 in late preconditioning. *Am. J. Physiol. Heart Circ. Physiol.* 279:H2269-H2276.

Oldenburg O, Cohen MV, Yellon DM, et al. (2002) Mitochondrial K(ATP) channels: role in cardioprotection. *Cardiovasc. Res.* 55:429-37.

Ovbiagele B, Kidwell CS, Starkman S, et al. (2003). Neuroprotective agents for the treatment of acute ischemic stroke. *Curr. Neurol. Neurosci. Rep.* 3:9 –20.

Oxman T, Arad M, Klein R, et al. (1997) Limb ischemia preconditions the heart against reperfusion tachyarrythmia. *Am. J. Physiol.* 273:H1707-12.

Pagliaro P, Gattullo D, Rastaldo R, et al. (2001) Ischemic preconditioning: from the first to the second window of protection. *Life Sci.*, 69:1-15.

Pain T, Yang XM, Critz SD, et al. (2000) Opening of mitochondrial K(ATP) channels triggers the preconditioned state by generating free radicals, *Circ. Res.* 87: 460-6.

Paratt JR (1994) Protection of the heart by ischemic preconditioning: mechanisms and possibilities for pharmacological expression. *Trends Pharmacol. Sci.* 15:19-25.

Parsons MW, Barber PA, Desmond PM, et al. (2002) Acute hyperglycemia adversely affects stroke outcome: a magnetic resonance imaging and spectroscopy study. *Ann. Neurol.* 52: 20–28.

Parsons M, Young L, Lee JE, et al. (2000) Distinct cardioprotective effects of adenosine mediated by differential coupling of receptor subtypes to phospholipases C and D. *FASEB J.* 14:1423-31.

Patel PM, Drummond JC, Cole DJ, et al. (1995). Isoflurane reduces ischemia-induced glutamate release in rats subjected to fore-brain ischemia. *Anesthesiology.* 82: 996–1003.

Perez-Pinzon MA, Dave KR, et al. (2005) Role of reactive oxygen species and protein kinase C in ischemic tolerance in the brain. *Antioxid. Redox Signal.* 7:1150-7.

Perez-Pinzon MA, Xu GP, Dietrich WD, et al. (1997) Rapid preconditioningn protects rats against ischemic neuronal damage after 3 but not 7 days of reperfusion following global cerebral ischemia. *J. Cereb. Blood Flow Metab.* 17:175-82.

Perkins ND (2000) The Rel/NF-kappa B family: friend and foe. *Trends Biochem. Sci.* 25: 434-40.

Pfenninger E, Himmelseher S (1997) Neuroprotection by ketamine at the cellular level. *Anaesthesist* 46:S47-S54.

Pike CJ, Vaughan PJ, Cuuningham DD, et al. (1996) Thrombin attenuates neuronal cell death and modulates astrocyte reactivity induced by beta-amyloid in vitro. *J. Neurochem.* 66:1374-82.

Ping P, Zhang J, Zheng YT, et al. (1999) Demonstration of selective protein kinase C-dependent activation of Src and Lck tyrosine kinases during ischemic preconditioning in conscious rabbits. *Circ. Res.* 85:542-50.

Ping P, Song C, Zhang J, et al. (2002) Formation of protein kinase C(epsilon)-Lck signaling modules confers cardioprotection. *J. Clin. Invest.* 109:499-507.

Post H, Heusch G (2002) Ischemic preconditioning. Experimental facts and clinical perspective. *Minerva Carioangiol* 50:569-605.

Prass K, Scharff A, Ruscher K, et al. (2003) Hypoxia-induced stroke tolerance in the mouse is mediated by erythropoietin. *Stroke.* 34:1981-6.

Prass K, Ruscher K, Karsch M, et al. (2002) Desferrioxamine induces delayed tolerance against cerebral ischemia in vivo and in vitro. *J. Cereb. Blood Flow Metab.* 22: 520–525.

Przyklenk K, Darling CE, Dickson EW, et al. (2003) Carioprotection "outsie the box" – evolving pardigm of remote preconditioning. *Basic Res. Cardiol.* 98:149-57.

Qin Q, Downey JM, Cohen MV (2003) Acetylcholine but not adenosine triggers preconditioning through PI3-kinase and a tyrosine kinase. *Am. J. Physiol. Heart Circ. Physiol.* 284:H727-34.

Quinlan JJ, Firestone S, Firestone LL (1995) Isoflurane's enhancement of chloride flux through rat brain?: aminobutyric acid type A receptors is stereoselective. *Anesthesiology.* 83: 611–615.Ravati A, Ahlemeyer B, Becker A, et al. (2000) Preconditioning-induced neuroprotection is mediated by reactive oxygen species, *Brain Res.* 866:23-32.

Ravati A, Ahelmeyer B, Becker A, et al. (2001) Preconditioning-induced neuroprotection is mediated by reactive oxygen species and activation of the transcription factor nuclear factor-kappaB. *J. Neurochem.*, 78:909-19.

Reimer KA, Murry CE, Yamasawa I, et al. (1986) Four brief periods of myocardial ischemia cuase no cumulative ATP loss or necrosis. *Am. J. Physiol.* 251:H-1306-15.

Reinoso-Suárez F. Topographischer Hirnatlas der Katze. Darmstadt, Germany: E Merck AG; 1961

Reivich M, Kuhl D, Wolf A, et al. (1979) The (18F) fluoordeoxyglucose method for the measurement of local cerebral glucose utliziation in man. *Circ. Res.* 44:127-137.

Reshef A, Sperling O, Zoref-Shani E. (2000) Role of K(ATP) channels in the induction of ischemic tolerance by the 'adenosine mechanism' in neuronal cultures. *Adv. Exp. Med. Biol.* 486:217-21.

Reshef A, Sperling O, Zoref-Shani E (2000a) The adenosine-induced mechanism for the acquisition of ischemic tolerance in primary rat neuronal cultures. *Pharmacol. Therapeut.*, 87: 151-159.

Reshef A, Sperling O, Zoref-Shani E (2000b) Opening of KATP channels is mandatory for acquisition of ischemic tolerance by adenosine. *Neuroreport,* 11: 463-465.

Reshef A, Sperling O, Shani E. (1998) Opening of ATP sensitive potassium channels by cromakalim confers tolerance against chemical ischemia in rat neuronal cultures, *Neurosci. Lett.,* 250:111-114.

Reshef A, Sperling O, Shani E (1997) Activation and inhibition of protein kinase C protect neuronal cultures against ischemia-reperfusion insult, *Neurosci. Lett.*, 238:37-40.

Reshef A, Sperling O., Shani E. (1996) Preconditioning of primary rat neuronal cultures against ischemic injury: characterization of the 'time window of protection'. *Brain Res.*, 741: 252-257.

Rheee SG, Bae YS (1997) Regulation of phosphoinositide-specific phospholipase C isozymes. *J. Biol. Chem.* 272:15045-8.

Rice ME, Forman RE, Chen BT, et al. Brain antioxidant regulation in mammals and anoxia-tolerant reptiles: balanced for neuroprotection and neuromodulation. *Comp. Biochem. Physiol. C Toxical. Pharmacol.* 133:515-25.

Richard V, Kaeffer N, Tron C, et al. (1994) Ischemic preconditioning protects against coronary endothelial dysfunction induced by ischemia and reperfusion. *Circulation.* 89:1254–1261.

Riepe MW, Kasischke K, Raupach A. (1997) Acetylsalicylic acid increases tolerance against hypoxic and chemical hypoxia. *Stroke*. 28:2006-11.

Riepe MW, Niemi WN, Megow D, et al. (1996) Mitochondrial oxidation in rat hippoamcpus can be precondtioninged by selective chemical inhibiion of usccinic dehydrogenase. *Exp. Neurol.* 138:15-21.

Ringelstein EB, Biniek R, Weiller C, et al. (1992) Type and extent of hemispheric brain infarctions and clinical outcome in early and delayed middle cerebral artery recanalization. *Neurology*. 42:289–298.

Rodrigo J, Fernandez AP, Serrano J, et al. (2005) The role of free radicals in cerebral hypoxia and ischemia. *Free Radic. Biol. Med.* 39:26-50.

Rogel A, Bromberg Y, Sperling O, et al. (2004) Phospholipase C is involved in the adenosine-activated signal transduction pathway conferring protection against iodoacetic acid-induced injury in primary rat neuronal cultures, *Neuroscience Letters*, in press.

Rohmann S, Weygandt H, Schelling,P, et al. (1994) Involvement of ATP-sensitive potassium channels in preconditioning protection, *Basic. Res. Cardiol.,* 89:563-576.

Rosner G, Graf R, Kataoka K, et al. (1986) Selective functional vulnerability of cortical neurons following transient MCA occlusion in the rat. *Stroke* 17:76-82.

Rothwell PM. (2003) Incidence, risk factors and prognosis of stroke and TIA: the need for high-quality, large-scale epidemiological studies and meta-analyses. *Cerebrovasc. Dis.* 16 (suppl 3): 2–10.

Rudolphi KA, Schubert P, Parkinson FE, et al. (1992) Neuroprotctive role of adenosine in cerebral ischemia, *Trends in Pharmacol. Sci.* 13:439-445.

Ruscher K, Freyer D, Karsch M, et al. (2002) Erythropoietin is a paracrine mediator of ischemic tolerance in the brain: evidence from an in vitro model. *J. Neurosci*. 22:10291–10301.

Saver JL, Kidwell C. (2004) Neuroimaging in TIAs. *Neurology*. 62: S22–S25.

Saver JL. (2004) Number needed to treat estimates incorporating effects over the entire range of clinical outcomes: novel derivation method and application to thrombolytic therapy for acute stroke. *Arch. Neurol*. 61:1066-70.

Schaller BJ, Buchfelder M. (2006) Neuroprotection in primary brain tumors: sense or nonsense? *Expert Rev. Neurother*. 6:723-30.

Schaller B (2005).Ischemic preconditioning as induction of ischemic tolerance after transient ischemic attacks in human brain: its clinical relevance. *Neurosci Lett*. 377:206-11.

Schaller B, Graf R, Sanada Y, et al. (2004) Decompressive hemicraniectomy in a new cat model. Methodological description of the PET study protocol. *Brain Res. Protocol.* 12:125-131.

Schaller B, Graf R. (2004) Cerebral ischemia and reperfusion: the pathophysiologic concept as a basis for clinical therapy. *J. Cereb. Blood Flow Metab.* 24:351-71.

Schaller B, Graf R, Jacobs AH. (2003) Ischaemic tolerance: a window to endogenous neuroprotection? *Lancet*. 362:1007.

Schaller B, Graf R, Sanada Y, et al. (2003) Hemodynamic and metabolic effects of decompressive hemicraniectomy in normal brain. An experimental PET-study in cats. *Brain Res*. 982:31-37.

Schaller B, Graf R (2003) Hypothermia and stroke: the pathophysiological background. *Pathophysiology* 10:7-35.

Schaller B, Graf R. (2002) Cerebral ischemic preconditioning. An experimental phenomenon or a clinical important entity of stroke prevention? *J. Neurol.* 249:1503-11.

Schipke JD, Halkos ME, Kerendi F, et al. (2006) Postconditioning. *Arch. Med. Sci.* 2:137-145.

Schwartz LM, Langranha CJ (2006) ischemic postconditioning during reperfusion activates Akt and ERK without proitecting against lethal myocardial ischemia-reperfusion injury in pigs. *Am. J. Physiol. Heart Circ. Physiol.* 290:H1011-8.

Schubert P, Rudolphi KA, Fedholm BB, et al. (1994) Modulation of nerve and glial function by adenosine - role in the development of ischemic damage, *Int. J. Biochem.* 6:1227-1236.

Schulte G, Fredholm BB (2003) Signalling from adenosine receptors to mitogen-activated protein kinases. *Cell. Signal.* 15:813-27.

Schulz R., Cohen MV, Behrends M., et al. (2001) Signal transduction of ischemic preconditioning. *Cardiovasc. Res.*, 52:181-98.

Semenza GL (2000) HIF-1: mediator of physiological and pathophysiological responses to hypoxia. *J. Appl. Physiol.* 88: 1474–1480.

Serviddio G, Di Venosa N, Federici A, et al. (2005) Brief hypoxia before normoxic reperfusion (postconditioning) protects the heart against ischemia-reperfusion injury by preventing mitochondria peroxide production and glutathione depletion. *FASEB J.* 19:354-61.

Shimazaki K, Nakamura K, Nakamura K, et al. (1998) Reduced calcium elevation in hippocampal CA1 neurons of ischemia tolerant gerbils. *Neuroreport* 9:1875-8.

Shimizu S, Nagayama T, Jin KL, et al. (2001) Bcl-2 antisense treatment prevents induction of tolerance to focal ischemia in the rat brain. *J. Cereb. Blood Flow Metab.* 21:233-43.

Shimohama S, Kihara T (2001) Nicotinic receptor-mediated protection against beta-amyloid neurotoxicity. *Biol. Psychiatry* 49:233-9.

Shou Y, Li N, Li L, et al. (2002) NF-kappaB-mediated up-regulation of Bcl-X(S) and Bax contributes to cytochrome c release in cyanide-induced apoptosis. *J. Neurochem.* 81: 842-52.

Shuaib A, Murabit M, Kanthan R, et al. (1996). The neuroprotective effects of gamma-vinyl GABA in transient global ischemia: a morphological study with early and delayed evaluations. *Neurosci. Lett.* 204: 1–4.

Shyu KG, Liang YJ, Chang H, et al. (2004) Enhanced expression of angiopoietin-2 and the tie2 receptor but not angiopoietin-1 or the tie1 receptor in a rat model of myocardial infarction. *J. Biomed. Sci.* 11:163-71.

Sicheri F, Kuriyan J (1997) Structures of Src-family tyrosine kinases. *Curr. Opin. Struct. Biol.* 7:777-85.

Simon RP, Niiro M, Gwinn R (1993) Prior ischemic stress protects agianst experimental stroke. *Neurosci. Lett.* 163:135-7.

Simon RP, Swan JH, Griffiths T, et al. (1984). Blockade of *N*-methyl-d-aspartate receptors may protect against ischemic damage in the brain. *Science* 226: 850–852.

Siren AL, Fratelli M, Brines M, et al. (2001) Erythropoietin prevents neuronal apoptosis after cerebral ischemia and metabolic stress. *Proc. Natl. Acad. Sci. USA* 98:4044-49.

Smith WS (2004) Pathophysiology of focal cerebral ischemia: a therapeutic perspective. *J. Vasc. Interv. Radiol.* 15:S3-12.

Spangenberger H, Nikmanesh FG, Igelmund P, et al. (1995) Effects of adenosine on synaptic transmission in hippocampal slices form hibernating and warm-acclimated Turkish hamersters and rats. *Neurosci. Lett.* 185:217-19.

Sperling O, Bromberg Y, Oelsner H, et al. (2003) Reactive oxygen species play an important role in iodoacetate-induced neurotoxicity in primary rat neuronal cultures and in differentiated PC12 cells, *Neurosci. Lett.* 351:137-140.

Stenzel-Poore MP, Stevens SL, Simon RP. (2004) Genomics of preconditioning. *Stroke* 35(11 Suppl 1):2683-6.

Stenzel-Poore MP, Stevens SL, Xiong Z, et al. (2003). Effect of ischemic preconditioning on genome response to cerebral ischemia: similarity to neuroprotective strategies in hibernation and hypoxia-tolerant states. *Lancet.* 362: 1028–1037.

Stagliano NE, Perez-Pinzon MA, Moskowitz MA, et al. (1999) Focal ischemic preconditioning induces rapid tolerance to middle cerebral artery occlusion in mice. *J. Cereb. Blood Flow Metab.* 19:757-61.

Storey KM, Storey J: (1990) Metabolic rate depression and biochemical adaptation in aneabiosis, hibernation and estivation. *Q Rev. Biol.* 65:145-74.

Striggow F, Riek M, Breder J, et al. (2000) The protease thrombin is an endogenous mediator of hippocampal neuroprotection against ischemia at low concentrations but causes degeneration at high concentrations. *Proc. Natl. Acad Sci. USA* 97:2264-9.

Stroke Therapy Academic Industry Roundtable (1999). STAIR. *Stroke* 30:2752-8.

Strong AJ, Venables GS, Gibson G (1983) The cortical ischaemic penumbra associated with occlusion of the middle cerebral artery in the cat. 1. Topography of changes in blood flow, potassium ion activity, and EEG. *J. Cereb. Blood Flow Metab.* 3:86-96.

Sydserff SG, Borelli AR, Green AR, et al. (2002). Effect of NXY-059 on infarct volume after transient or permanent middle cerebral artery occlusion in the rat: studies on dose, plasma concentration and therapeutic time window. *Br. J. Pharmacol.* 135: 103–112.

Swain JL, Sabina RL, Hines JJ, et al. (1984) Repetitive episodes of brief ischemia (12 minutes) do not produce a cumulative depletion of high-energy phosphate compounds. *Cardiovasc Res* 18:264-9.

Swartz KL (1993) Modulation of Ca^{2+} channels by protein kinase C in rat central and peripheral neurons: disruption of G protein mediated inhibition, *Neuron.*, 11:305-320.

Taguchi A, Soma T, Tanaka H, et al (2004). Administration of CD34+ cells after stroke enhances neurogenesis via angiogenesis in a mouse model. *J. Clin. Invest.* 114: 330–338.

Takaoka A, Nakae I, Mitsunami K, et al. (1999). Renal ischemia/reperfusion remotely improves myocardial energy metabolism during myocardial ischemia via adenosine receptors in rabbits: effects of "remote preconditioning." *J. Am. Coll Cardiol.* 33:556–564.

Takayama K, Suzuki T, Miura M. (1994) The comparison of effects of various anesthetics on expression of Fos protein in the rat brain. *Neurosci. Lett.* 173: 59–62.

Takano H, Manchikalapudi S, Tang XL, et al. (1998) Nitric oxide synthase is the mediator of late preconditioning against myocardial infarction in conscious rabbits. *Circulation.* 98: 441–449.

Takeda A, Onodera H, Sugimoto A, et al. (1993). Coordinated expression of messenger RNAs for nerve growth factor, brain-derived neurotrophic factor and neurotophin-3 in the rat hippocampus following transient forebrain ischemia. *Neuroscience.* 55:23–31.

Taylor CP, Meldrum BS (1995) Na+ channels as targets for neuroprotective drugs. *Trends Pharmacol Sci* 16 :309 –316.

The National Institute of Neurological Disorders and Stroke rt-PA Stroke Study Group (1995) Tissue plasminogen activator for acute ischemic stroke. *N. Engl. J. Med.* 333:1581 –1587.

Thourani VH, Nakamura M, Duarte IG, et al. (1999) Ischemic preconditioning attenuates postischemic coronary artery endothelial dysfunction in a model of minimally invasive direct coronary bypass grafting. *J. Thorac. Cardiovasc. Surg.* 117:383–389.

Todd JC, Zhao ZQ, Williams MW, et al. (1996) Intravascular adenosine at reperfusion reduces infarct size and eutrophil adherence. *Ann. Thorac. Surg.* 62:1364-72.

Todd JC, Williams MW, Zhao ZQ, et al. Polyadenylic adcid reduces infarct size via intravascualr adenosine recpetor mechanism during reperufsion. *FASEB J.* 9:A421 (Abstract).

Togashi H, Sasaki M, Frohman E, et al. (1997). Neuronal (type I) nitric oxide synthase regulates nuclear factor kappaB activity and immunologic (type II) nitric oxide synthase expression. *Proc. Natl. Acad. Sci. USA.* 94: 2676–2680.

Tomai F, Crea F, Chaireillo L, et al. (1999) Ischemic preconditioning in humans: models, mediators, and clinical relevance. *Circulation* 74:1124-36.

Toyoda T, Kassell NF, Lee KS (1997) Induction of ischemic tolerance and antioxidant activity by brief focal ischemia. *Neuroreport* 8:847-51.

Toullec D, Pianetti P, Coste H, et al. (1991) The bisindolylmaleimide GF 109203X is a potent and selective inhibitor of protein kinase C, *J. Biol. Chem.*, 266:15771-81.

Trendelenburg G, Dirnagl U.(2005) Neuroprotective role of astrocytes in cerebral ischemia: focus on ischemic preconditioning. *Glia.* 50:307-20.

Tsang A, Hausenloy DJ, Mocanu MM, et al. (2004) Postconditioning: a form of "modified reperfusion" protects the myocardium by activating the phosphatidyliniositol 3-kinase-Akt pathway. *Circ. Res.* 95:230-2.

Vahlhaus C, Schulz R, Post H, et al. (1998) Prevention of ischemic preconditioning only by combined inhibition of protein kinase C and protein tyrosine kinase in pigs. *J. Mol. Cell. Cardiol.* 30:197-209.

Valentim LM, Geyer AB, Tavares A, et al. (2001) Effects of global cerebral ischemia and preconditioning on heat shock protein 27 immunocontent and phosphorylation in rat hippocampus. *Neuroscience* 107:43-9.

Vass K, Tomida S, Hossmann KA, et al. (1988) Microvascular disturbances and edema formation after repetitive ischemia of gerbil brain. *Acta Neuropathol. (Berl)* 75:288-94.

Vigh L, Literati PN, Horvath I, et al (1997) A non-toxic, hyodrxylamine deprivate with stress protein-inducring activity and cytoprotective effects. *Nature Med.* 3:1150-54.

Vinen-Johansen J, Zaho ZQ, Zatta AJ, et al. (2005) Postconditioning – a new link in nature`s armor against myocardial ischemia-reperfusion injury. *Basics Res. Cardiol.* 100:295-310.

Vondriska TM, Zhang J, Song C, et al. (1998) Protein kinase C epsilon-Src moduoes direct signal transduction in nitric oxide-induced cardioprotection: complex ofrmation as a means for cardioprotective signaling. *Circ. Res.* 88:1306-13.

Walton MR, Dragunow I (2000) Is CREB a key to neuronal survival? *Trends Neurosci.* 23:48-53.

Wann KT (1993) Neuronal sodium and potassium channels: structure and function. *Br. J. Anaesth* 71:2-14.

Warner DS, McFarlane C, Todd MM, et al. (1993) Sevoflurane and halothane reduce focal ischemic brain damage in the rat: possible influence on thermoregulation. *Anesthesiology.* 79:985–992.

Wassmann H, Greiner C, Hulsmann S, et al. (1998) Hypothermia as cerebroprotective measure: experimental hypoxic exposure of brain slices and clinical application in critically reduced cerebral perfusion pressure. *Neurol. Res.* 20(suppl 1) :S61 –65.

Watson BD, Prado R, Veloso A, et al. (2002). Cerebral blood flow restoration and reperfusion injury after ultraviolet laser-facilitated middle cerebral artery recanalization in rat thrombotic stroke. *Stroke* 33 :428 –434.

Weber NC, Preckel B, Schlack W (2005) The effect of anaesthetics on the myocardium – new insights into myocardial protection. *Eur. J. Anaesthesiol.* 22:647-57.

Wei L, Erinjeri JP, Rovainen CM, et al. (2001). Collateral growth and angiogenesis around cortical stroke. *Stroke* 32: 2179–2184.

Weih M, Prass K, Ruscher K, et al. (2001) Ischemic tolerance. Modell for the research, hope for the clinic? *Nervenarzt* 72:255-260.

Weih M, Kallenberg K, Bergk A, et al. (1999) Attenuated stroke severity after prodromal TIA: a role for ischemic tolerance in the brain? *Stroke* 30:1851-4.

Wick A, Wick W, Waltenberger J, et al. (2002) Neuroprotetion by hypoxic preconditioning requires sequential activation of vascular endothelial growth factor receptor and Akt. *J. Neurosci.* 22:6401-7.

Widmann R, Kuroiwa T, Bonnekoh P, et al. (1991) Leucine incorporation into brain proteins in erbils after transient ischemia: relationsship to selective vulnerability of hippocampus. *J. Neurochem.* 56:789-96.

Wiegand F, Liao W, Busch C, et al. (1999) Respiratory chain inhibition induces tolerance to focal cerebral ischemia. *J. Cereb. Blood Flow Metab.* 19:1229-37.

Wienhard K, Dahlbom M, Eriksson L, et al. (1994) The ECAT EXACT HR: performance of a new high resolution positron scanner. *J. Comput. Assist. Tomogra* 18:110-118.

Wienhard K, Pawlik G, Herholz K, et al. (1985) Estimation of local cerebral utilizaition by positron emission tomography fo (18F)-2-fluoro-2-deoxy-D-glucose: a critical appraisal of optimization procedures. *J. Cereb. Blood Flow Metab.* 5:115-125.

Wong GH, Goeddel DV (1988) Induction of manganous superoxide dismutase by tumor necrosis factor: possible protective mechanism. *Science* 242:941-4.

Xi G, Hua Y, Keep R, et al. (2000) Induction of colligin may attenuate brain edema following intracerebral hemorrhage. *Acta Neurochir.* 76:501-505.

Xi G, Keep RF, Hua Y, et al. (1999) Attenuation of thrombin-induced brain edema by central thrombin preconditioning. *Stroke* 30:1247-55.

Yagita Y, Kitagawa K, Ohtsuki T, et al. (2001) Induction of the HSP110/105 family in the rat hippocmapus in the cerebral ischemia and ischemic tolerance. *J. Cereb. Blood Flow Metab.* 21:811-9.

Yang J, Zorumski CF (1991) Effects of isoflurane on N-methyl-D-aspartate gated ion channels in cultured rat hippocampal neurons. *Ann. N Y Acad. Sci.* 625: 287–289.

Yavin Z, Yavin E (1977) Synaptogenesis and myelingenesis in dissocated cerebral cells from rat embryo on polylysine coated surfaces. *Exp. Brain Res.* 29:137-47.

Yedovitzkiy M, Mochly-rosen D, Johnson JA, et al. (1997) Translocation inhibitors define specifity of protein kinase C isoenzymes in pancreatic beta-cells. *J. Biol. Chem.* 272:1417-20.

Yenari MA; Fink SL, Sun GH, et al. (1998) Gene therapy with Hsp 72 is neuroprotecitve in rat models of stroke and epilepsy. *Ann. Neurol.* 44:584-91.

Yewdell JW (2001) Not such a dismal sience: the economics of protein synthesis, folding degration and antigen processing. *Trends Cell Biol.* 11:294-7.

Yoneda Y, Azuma Y, Inoue K, et al (1997). Positive correlation between prolonged potentiation of binding of double-stranded oligonucleotide probe for the transcription factor AP1 and resistance to transient forebrain ischemia in gerbil hippocampus. *Neuroscience* 79: 1023–1037.

Yu ZF, Mattson MP (1999) Dietary restriction and 2-deoxyglucose administration reduce focal ischemic brain damage and improve behavioural outcome: evidence for a preconditioning mechanism. *J. Neurosci Res.* 57:830-839.

Yu ZF, Bruce-Keller AJ, Goodman Y, et al. (1998). Uric acid protects neurons against excitotoxic and metabolic insults in cell culture, and against focal ischemic brain injury in vivo. *J. Neurosci. Res.*; 53: 613–625.

Zhao H, Sapolsky RM, Steinberg GK (2006) Interrupting reperfusion as a stroke therapy: ischemic postconditioning reduces infarct size after focal ischemia in rats. *J. Cereb. Blood Flow Metab.* 26:1114-21.

Zhao ZQ, Corvera JS; Halkos ME, et al. Inhibition of myocardial injury by ischemic postconditioning during reperfusion: comparison with ischemic preconditioning. *Am. J. Physiol. Heart Circ. Physiol.* 285:H579-88.

Zhan RZ, Fujihara H, Baba H, et al. (2002) Ischemic preconditioningn is capable of inducing mitochondrial tolerance in the rat brain. *Anesthsiology* 97:896-901.

Zoref-Shani E, Bromberg Y, Lilling G, et al. (1995) Development changes in purine nucleotide metabolism in cultured rat astroglia. *Int. J. Developmental Neuroscience* 13:887-896.

Index

A

D

E

O

P

R

S

T